GW01271354

CONTENTS

WELCOME

Less stress, inner calm, more happiness and better health. Sounds good? These are just some of the rewards that mindfulness can bring. If you've heard the buzz about this ancient practice but aren't sure what it is or where to start, *The Mindfulness Workbook* is the guide you need. Forget about hours of sitting in the lotus position, trying to empty your mind. At its simplest, mindfulness is about becoming more present and living fully in the moment. If you've found yourself pausing to appreciate the beauty of a sunset, breathing in the smell of freshly cut grass on a summer's day or feeling a sense of serenity at the end of a yoga class, you've experienced mindfulness.

In *The Mindfulness Handbook*, you'll find step-by-step exercises and expert advice to help you develop this beneficial state of mind and apply your new skills to daily life. Whether you want to beat work stress, deepen your relationships, boost your wellbeing or feel more joy, you're now on the path to a happier, richer life.

HOW TO USE THIS BOOK

1. Learn the basics P10
Mindfulness might be an ancient practice but research is proving it has many benefits for modern-day life. Start here to discover exactly what mindfulness is, the science behind it and how it can help you. You'll also experience your first five minutes of mindfulness practice.

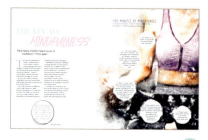

4. Apply your skills P66
Now you've learnt the basics, it's time to apply your new-found knowledge to daily life. Learn how to be a calmer commuter and beat work stress using just your reath, enjoy more mindful mealtimes and create a harmonious family life with just a few mindfulness tips.

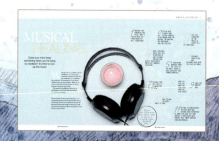

Keen to start reaping the benefits of mindfulness? Read these instructions first to get the most out of your guide

2. Move into mindfulness

It's time to start taking your first steps to becoming more mindful. Learn how to slow down your life and remove distractions. Try a couple of easy but effective mindfulness exercises and complete the first few entries in your 28-day Mindfulness Journal.

3. Master meditation

The art of meditation is a key way to enrich your mindfulness practice – and it's not as hard as you think! Discover how mindfulness meditation can change your brain for the better; learn the foundations and try some simple meditation techniques, including one that can spread the power of happiness.

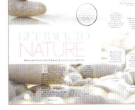

5. Get moving

Still finding it hard to relax your mind or find a few minutes to meditate? It's time to try mindfulness on the move. Science shows that getting active can help focus your mind and so, in this section, you'll find a selection of moving meditations to try – from mindful walking and running to a soothing yoga session.

6. Heal yourself

The healing powers of mindfulness are many and, in this final section, we let you into the secrets. Discover how bringing back play and laughter into your life can boost your health, why trying a craft could be your route to happiness, and how to conjure up your ideal life.

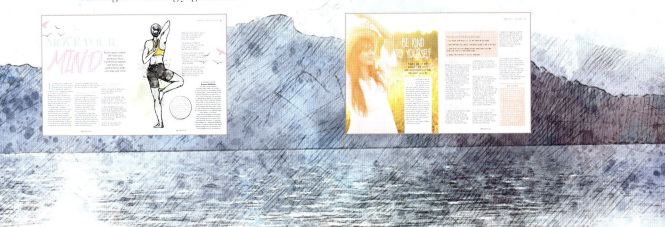

'Do not dwell in the past,
do not dream of the future,
concentrate the mind on
the present moment.'

BUDDHA

THE BASICS

Heard about the benefits of mindfulness but not sure exactly what it is? Prepare to discover how this simple, ancient practice can transform your life, health and happiness. First, you'll learn about the history and foundations of mindfulness. Then, read about its many science-backed benefits, from boosting brain power to reducing pain. Find out how naturally mindful you are and try a simple five-minute mindfulness exercise. Read on to begin your journey.

INTRODUCTION TO
MINDFULNESS

Mindfulness is the buzzword of the moment. But behind the wellbeing trend lies a profoundly life-changing philosophy. Here's what you need to know

Ever reached for your morning cuppa only to notice it's already empty? Or driven from A to B only to realise you didn't register much of the journey? It's called living on autopilot. We're so preoccupied with to-do lists and juggling a multitude of tasks that, before we know it, our days have merged into an endless check-list and we rarely have time to enjoy just being. This means we miss out on so much - not just the beauty of a sunset or the smile of a stranger, but the sense of calm and ease that comes from being mindful.

Simply by being fully present, aware of your thoughts, emotions and bodily sensations, you are able to inhabit the moment in a way that brings a

Mindfulness has become a huge trend, used in almost every walk of life from health to education. But it's easy to learn - you don't even need to attend a class.

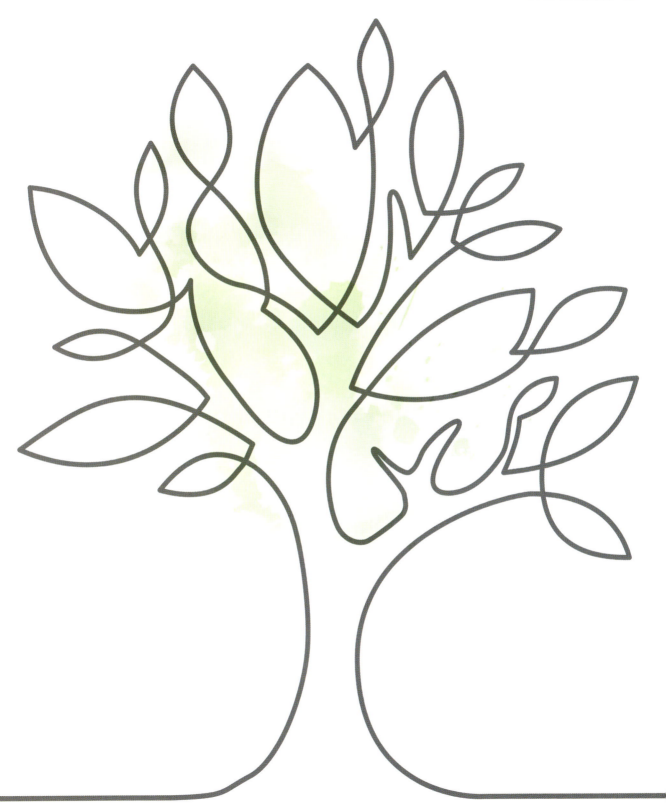

HOW MINDFUL ARE YOU?

Being mindful equals being present. Check out if you could be more mindful by answering these questions:

1 If you feel sad or disappointed, do you allow yourself to fully experience your feelings?

2 Do you notice your thoughts as if you're observing them from the outside – that is, without identifying with them?

3 When faced with an unexpected event – pleasant or unpleasant – are you aware of how your body responds?

4 When your mood changes, are you aware of the thoughts that may have contributed to the way you feel now?

5 Are you aware of what you are feeling at the time?

wealth of benefits, including less stress, better communication, more satisfying relationships and increased focus. It's even been shown to enhance your immune system.

THE ORIGINS

Mindfulness has its roots in the early religious teachings of the Eastern world, particularly Buddhism. However, mindfulness as we know it today was developed by an American scientist called Jon Kabat-Zinn. Back in the 1970s, he discovered that Buddhist meditation techniques had surprising results for wellbeing.

In one study, Kabat-Zinn taught patients with skin disorders to focus on the present moment while receiving ultra-violet light treatment, and found their conditions cleared up four times the rate of the non-meditators.

The results of his research were so impressive, he went on to develop an eight-week stress-reduction programme called Mindfulness-Based Stress Reduction (MBSR) which forms the basis of many mindfulness courses today.

MODERN-DAY MINDFULNESS

Nowadays mindfulness tends to be practiced in two ways.

● Many people begin with formal practices, where you set aside time to sit and meditate or follow a specific mindfulness practice such as the body scan (p52) or mindful eating (p76).

● You can also develop a more general mindful way of being throughout your day by bringing your attention to the present moment and becoming completely absorbed in it – switching from 'doing mode' to 'being mode' no matter what you are doing.

Whether you're practising yoga, preparing supper, working on an intense project or sitting on a train, being fully aware of the moment will make the experience richer, more fulfilling and good for your health.

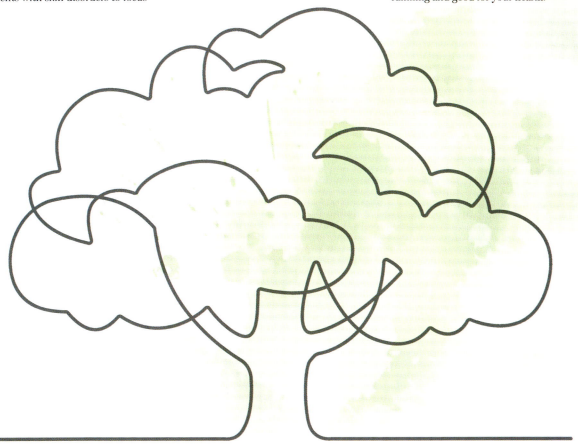

THE KEY TO
MINDFULNESS

Think being mindful means hours of meditation? Think again…

The secret of mindfulness is simple – paying attention to the moment. It doesn't mean emptying your mind of thoughts or sitting in the lotus position and meditating. By simply being fully present and 'spacious' – aware of your thoughts, emotions and senses without getting caught up in them – you can reap a wealth of benefits including less stress and anxiety, better relationships and creativity and improved focus and self esteem.

One of the key reasons mindfulness works is that it opens up a space between what happens to you and how you react. This means you can choose how to act in daily situations, rather than falling into unconscious patterns of behaviour that may be damaging.

'Mindfulness is awareness, cultivated by paying attention in a sustained and particular way; on purpose, in the present moment and non-judgementally,' says Jon Kabat-Zinn. 'This kind of attention nurtures greater awareness, clarity and acceptance of present-moment reality. If we're not fully present for many of these moments, we fail to realise the richness and depth of our possibilities for growth and transformation.'

Learning to live mindfully in the here and now, helps you to live a deeper, more balanced and satisfying existence, with more appreciation, wonder, empathy for others and, above all, greater self-understanding and ease.

By allowing you to appreciate the smaller moments in life, mindfulness can bring a great sense of calm to your daily life.

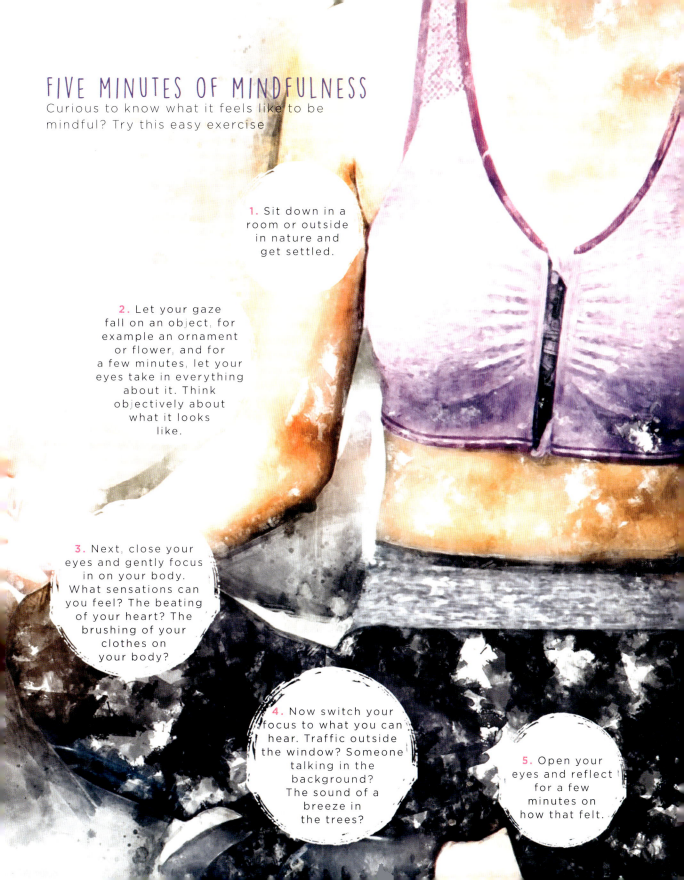

FIVE MINUTES OF MINDFULNESS

Curious to know what it feels like to be mindful? Try this easy exercise

1. Sit down in a room or outside in nature and get settled.

2. Let your gaze fall on an object, for example an ornament or flower, and for a few minutes, let your eyes take in everything about it. Think objectively about what it looks like.

3. Next, close your eyes and gently focus in on your body. What sensations can you feel? The beating of your heart? The brushing of your clothes on your body?

4. Now switch your focus to what you can hear. Traffic outside the window? Someone talking in the background? The sound of a breeze in the trees?

5. Open your eyes and reflect for a few minutes on how that felt.

SOUND
SLEEP

SELF
CONFIDENCE

NEW MIND
NEW YOU

Living in the moment
brings a wealth of benefits
for body and mind….

REDUCED
STRESS

IMPROVED
MEMORY

FASTER
BRAIN

HAPPIER
MIND

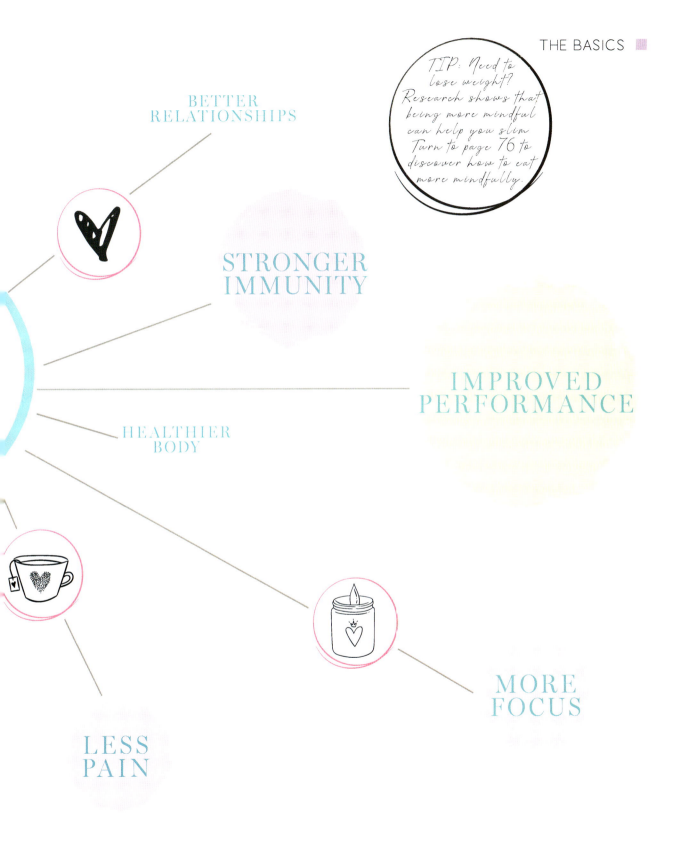

TIP: Need to lose weight? Research shows that being more mindful can help you slim. Turn to page 76 to discover how to eat more mindfully.

BETTER
RELATIONSHIPS

STRONGER
IMMUNITY

IMPROVED
PERFORMANCE

HEALTHIER
BODY

MORE
FOCUS

LESS
PAIN

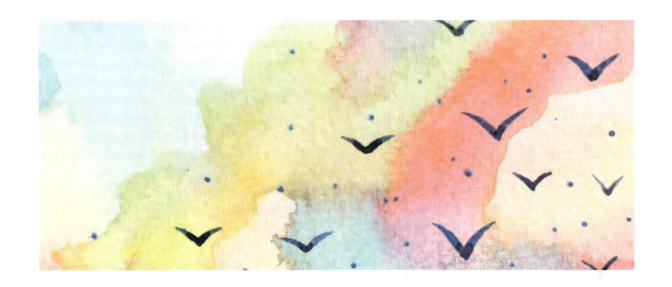

MINDFUL
BENEFITS

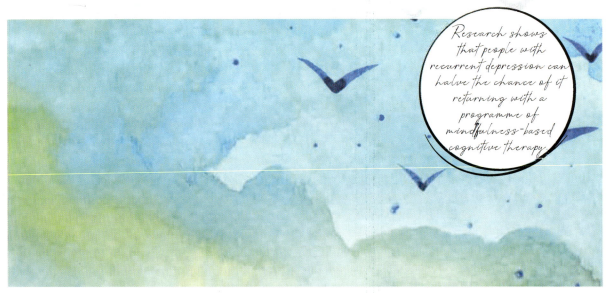

Research shows that people with recurrent depression can halve the chance of it returning with a programme of mindfulness-based cognitive therapy.

Mindfulness doesn't just make you feel calmer, it has many other powers too. Read on to discover more

You probably think of mindfulness as a way to relax and de-stress. But did you know that being mindful can help reduce pain and prevent illness? That it can make you more creative and better at making decisions? Or boost your happiness and even ease clinical depression? These are just some of the incredible findings that are being uncovered by science. Here are a few of the benefits you can expect to enjoy.

REDUCE PAIN

Suffering from chronic pain? Mindfulness is proven to help. Research funded by the National Institutes of Health in the US, showed mindfulness meditation relieves chronic pain more effectively than medical treatments. And it's not just psychological – mindfulness can physically reduce pain by altering activity in the brain.

In a study published in *The Journal of Neuroscience*, scientists found that people who were more mindful had less activity in a brain network that registers pain. 'Based on our research, we know we can increase mindfulness through relatively short periods of mindfulness meditation training,' said researcher Fadal Zeidan, 'So this may prove an effective way to provide pain relief.'

EASE DEPRESSION

Want to lift the blues? Mindfulness is an effective treatment to reduce clinical depression and improve mood. Neuroscientists have discovered it activates an area of the brain – the left

pre-frontal cortex – associated with positive emotions. When neuroscientist Professor Richard Davidson at the University of Wisconsin, USA, scanned the brains of regular meditators (including Buddhist monks), he discovered they have higher activation on the left side of their brains. And research at Oxford University shows mindfulness-based cognitive therapy (MCBT) is as effective as medication for preventing recurrent depression. With its focus on the present moment, mindfulness nurtures contentment and happiness.

Want to heal and enrich your relationship with yourself and others? Practise the loving kindness meditation (p60) once a week.

BOOST YOUR BRAIN

Struggling to learn a new language or make decisions at work? Take time out for some mindfulness. One recent German study showed that 10 minutes of mindfulness meditation a day improves concentration and working memory. From studying brain scans, the scientists found that mindfulness makes the brain more efficient at processing information, requiring fewer resources to do tasks. It also improves your decision-making powers and helps you learn to filter out distractions to focus on the task in hand.

IMPROVE RELATIONSHIPS

By teaching you greater awareness, compassion and acceptance of

yourself and others, mindfulness can strengthen and enrich your relationships. But it also works on a physiological level – research shows that mindfulness strengthens an area of the brain associated with cognitive flexibility, improving your ability to see problems from a different perspective.

It also calms an area of the brain that perceives threat, helping you react with judgement rather than from the heat of your emotions. This makes it easier to step back from conflict, stave off negative emotions, such as jealousy, communicate your feelings more honestly, and develop more meaningful bonds. Meditation also activates part of the brain that plays a key role in empathy – a key ingredient for love and compassion.

LOVE YOURSELF

Plagued by insecurities? Mindful meditation is a fast-track to greater self worth and confidence. By helping you become aware of negative self-talk and observe your thoughts in a non-judgemental way, mindfulness can turn the downward spiral of self-doubt into a positive cycle of self esteem. In one study, scientists found that people who were given meditation training saw a significant reduction in body-confidence insecurities and an increased appreciation of their bodies, within just three weeks.

'The little things? The little moments? They aren't little'

JON KABAT-ZINN

MOVING INTO MINDFULNESS

It's time to take your first steps to becoming more mindful. In this section,
you'll learn how to slow down and connect to the moment. Try a simple
breathing meditation you can use whenever you need to calm
down, and learn easy ways to switch from 'doing' to 'being' mode.
You can also complete the first few pages of your 28-day
Mindfulness Journal, specially designed to help support
your mindfulness journey. Try the daily tips and exercises,
and jot down how you're feeling and your
favourite mindful moments.

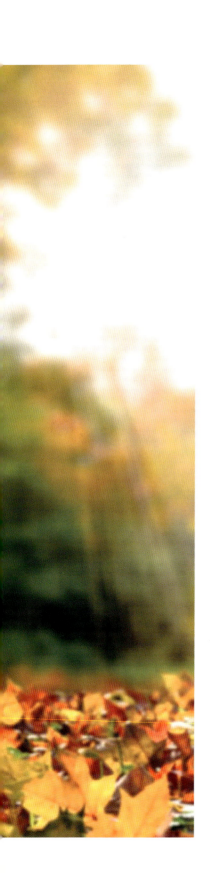

JUST BE

Want to become more mindful? It's time to switch from 'doing' to 'being'

Modern life is all about doing. Never-ending to-do lists to tick off, work deadlines to meet, family holidays to organise. Even when we think we're relaxing, our mind is typically planning ahead, worrying about upcoming situations or what people think of us, or cogitating over events in the recent past. Sounds familiar? No wonder stress is on the rise.

Learning to step away from this pattern of behaviour, to 'be' rather than 'do', is central to achieving mindfulness. To step into 'being' mode means focusing on the present moment without engaging with thoughts of the past or future, or reacting to distractions and emotions that arise. So, for instance on your walk to work, rather than mentally rehearsing your day, focus on the sights and sounds around you, whether it's the dewy roses and scent of freshly cut grass in the park, or the architectural shapes of buildings you pass in the street. When other thoughts arise, simply acknowledge them as a thought and refocus.

As you can imagine, 'being' takes some practice. But once you start, the feeling is so rewarding, you'll want to continue. And, with the help of exercises, such as the ones you'll find in this book, this mindful behaviour will start to come more naturally.

Sweeping leaves is a classic Buddhist mindfulness practice. As you sweep, focus on the rhythm of your body sweeping and the leaves rustling, letting all other thoughts float away.

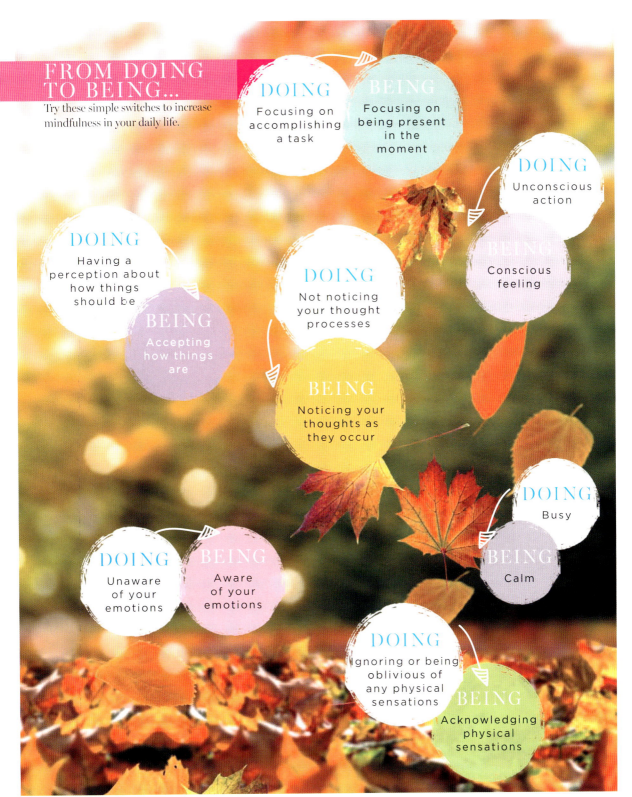

FROM DOING TO BEING...

Try these simple switches to increase mindfulness in your daily life.

DOING — Focusing on accomplishing a task

BEING — Focusing on being present in the moment

DOING — Unconscious action

BEING — Conscious feeling

DOING — Having a perception about how things should be

BEING — Accepting how things are

DOING — Not noticing your thought processes

BEING — Noticing your thoughts as they occur

DOING — Busy

BEING — Calm

DOING — Unaware of your emotions

BEING — Aware of your emotions

DOING — Ignoring or being oblivious of any physical sensations

BEING — Acknowledging physical sensations

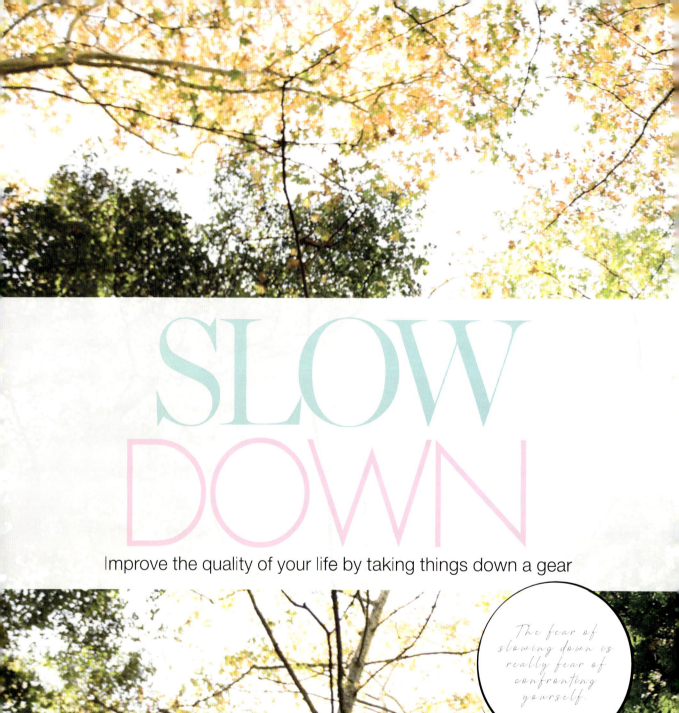

SLOW DOWN

Improve the quality of your life by taking things down a gear

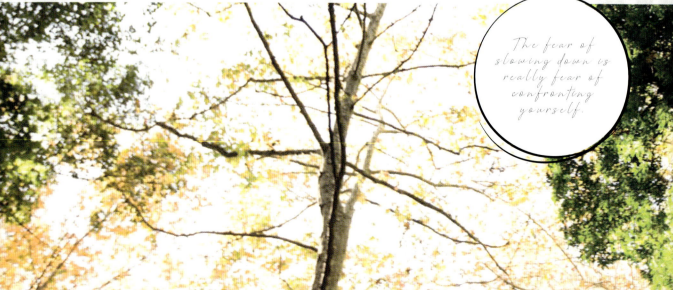

The fear of slowing down is really fear of confronting yourself.

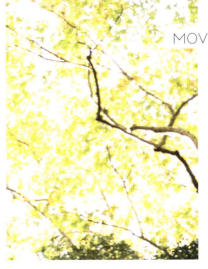

Our obsession with living life in the fast lane means that we often race through life instead of actually living or experiencing it. Everything suffers – our health, diet and relationships. We make mistakes at work, we can't relax or enjoy the moment, and we find it hard to sleep.

The antidote? It's time to follow the example of the growing Slow Movement and take time to enjoy the things that really give you pleasure. 'The secret is balance,' says Carl Honore in his book In Praise of Slow (Orion Books, £8.99). 'Instead of doing everything faster, do everything at the right speed. Sometimes fast, sometimes slow. Sometimes somewhere in between.'

It's not about rejecting modern-day life but simply changing gear every now and then to reconnect with food, people and places and create a more enjoyable life. To bring your shoulders down from around your ears, stop swearing at other drivers and bring your stressed-out pace down a little – even if it's just for an hour a day.

It can be as easy as switching off your mobile phone or tablet and sitting on a park bench watching the world go by for half an hour, or cooking with some fresh herbs for a change.

THINK ABOUT THE FOLLOWING:

● If 100 miles an hour is the top speed in your engine – what speed do you usually travel at? What would have to change in your life to slow down? More childcare? More support at work? More help at home?

● What are you trying to prove by living your life so fast?

● When during your day/week/year would be a good time to change gear and try a different pace?

● How can you service your engine to make 'slow' feel as powerful as 'fast'? For example, are your 'slow' times when you are most creative or sleep the most soundly? How can you increase the currency of slow?

3 WAYS TO SLOW DOWN

TAKE AN HOUR

Make sure you keep a date with yourself and take an hour to slow down. Think about how you'll use your slow hour. Will you be able to relax, rather than ticking things off your to-do list?

NOT TOO FAST

Don't slow down too quickly. If you're a rush-aholic, the first impulse may be to try too hard and expect instant results. Making a change takes time and isn't always easy. Plan it in increments.

PAY ATTENTION

Focus! Slowing down helps you give full attention to what you're doing and helps you find your flow. Walk at a slower pace, pause before speaking, and speak more slowly.

Day 1

GET AN IDEA OF THE MEANING OF MINDFULNESS BY PAYING FULL ATTENTION TO YOUR BREATHING FOR JUST ONE MINUTE. BE AWARE OF THE AIR AGAINST THE INSIDE OF YOUR NOSTRILS AS YOU INHALE. FEEL THE MOVEMENT OF YOUR CHEST AS IT BEGINS TO EXPAND AND THE BEAT OF YOUR HEART. NOW, FEEL YOUR BREATH AGAIN AS YOU EXHALE, AND THE FALL OF YOUR CHEST AS IT CONTRACTS (SEE P30 FOR MORE ADVICE.)

HOW I FELT

TODAY'S MINDFUL MOMENTS

Day 2

GAZE OUT OF THE WINDOW. MOST OF US SPEND ALL OUR TIME 'DOING' RATHER THAN 'BEING'. TODAY, LET YOURSELF SIT QUIETLY AND LOOK OUT OF THE WINDOW FOR FIVE MINUTES. WHEN YOUR MIND STARTS THINKING ABOUT SOMETHING – WHICH IT WILL – GENTLY BRING IT BACK TO THE PRESENT MOMENT.

HOW I FELT

TODAY'S MINDFUL MOMENTS

Day 3

STOP MULTI—TASKING! JUST FOR TODAY — OR EVEN FOR AN HOUR — AVOID JUGGLING HALF
A DOZEN TASKS AND CONCENTRATE ON FINISHING ONE ACTIVITY BEFORE MOVING ONTO THE
NEXT. FOCUS ON EVERY DETAIL OF THE JOB AND COMPLETE IT PROPERLY. NOTICE HOW IT
FEELS TO IMMERSE YOURSELF TOTALLY IN AN ACT FROM START TO FINISH, COMPARED WITH
SPREADING YOURSELF THIN. NOT ONLY WILL IT BOOST YOUR MINDFULNESS, RESEARCH SHOWS
WE'RE ACTUALLY MORE PRODUCTIVE WHEN WE MONO—TASK.

HOW I FELT

TODAY'S MINDFUL MOMENTS

BE FOCUSED, GET HAPPY

Too much going on to have a mindful moment? Here's how to reduce the distractions in your life

Do you constantly find yourself doing more but getting less done? Just as you're about to start on an important project at work, the phone rings. While you're answering it, a text pings in and meanwhile, the emails are piling up. Being bombarded with distractions is bad for us – it takes us away from the present moment, meaning we're not fully living our lives. It's mentally draining and can make you forget to do important things. Try these tips to help you stay focused, make the most of your time, and avoid losing touch with the things that are most precious to you.

1 TAKE A TECH BREAK

At work and at home, allow yourself time away from computers and phones. Switch them off altogether for a specific time period. Being available to respond to people's queries and requests all the time means you're constantly half-expecting the phone to ring or an email to arrive so you can neither relax nor get the time to fully engage with the task at hand.

2 FOCUS ON LIFE AT THE START AND END OF YOUR DAY

avoiding computers, phones and TV screens for the first hour of your waking day. Engaging with real life for a healthier start and end to the day, encouraging to be more focused

3 MAKE A GOAL

4 SET YOUR PRIORITIES

5 PROTECT YOUR TIME

MINDFUL
BREATHING

This five-minute exercise is one of
the cornerstones of mindfulness

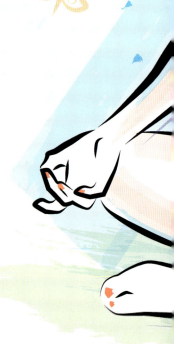

One of the simplest introductions to mindfulness is mindful breathing. It's an easy way to connect to the moment. You can do this anywhere – at home, in the office or on your commute to work. Bringing your attention to your breath can change everything. It brings you back to your true self and what you're feeling in the moment.

When we're stressed, busy or tired, our breath can become shallow, triggering a cycle of stress. Physically, taking a moment to connect with and deepen your breath helps oxygenate your body and calm your mind, even reducing blood pressure and relieving tension headaches.

Practise this exercise regularly, and you'll become more aware of how you breathe and make it easier to sink into deeper breathing at will.

1. Sit down in a comfortable position, such as cross legged. If you're sitting in a chair, keep your feet flat on the floor and your legs uncrossed. Relax your shoulders and keep your back straight. Rest your hands on your legs.

2. Close your eyes or lower your gaze.

3. Allow your body to relax and your mind to feel settled.

4. Breathe in through your nose and exhale through

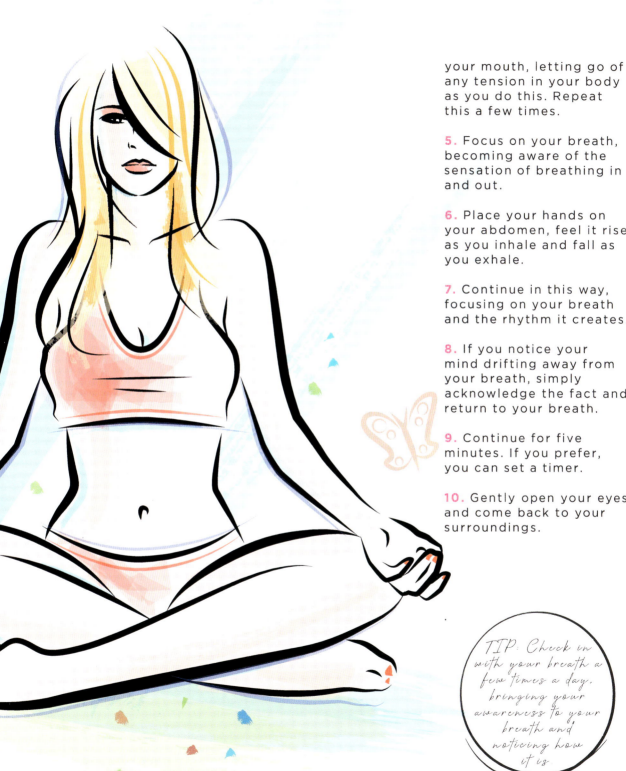

your mouth, letting go of any tension in your body as you do this. Repeat this a few times.

5. Focus on your breath, becoming aware of the sensation of breathing in and out.

6. Place your hands on your abdomen, feel it rise as you inhale and fall as you exhale.

7. Continue in this way, focusing on your breath and the rhythm it creates.

8. If you notice your mind drifting away from your breath, simply acknowledge the fact and return to your breath.

9. Continue for five minutes. If you prefer, you can set a timer.

10. Gently open your eyes and come back to your surroundings.

TIP: Check in with your breath a few times a day, bringing your awareness to your breath and noticing how it is.

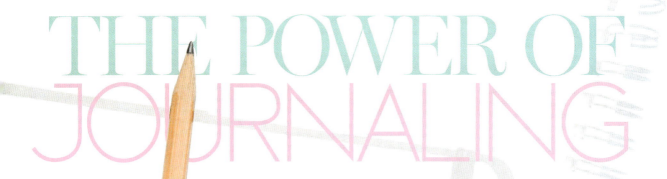

THE POWER OF
JOURNALING

Want to calm your mind
and heal your body? All you
need is a pen and paper

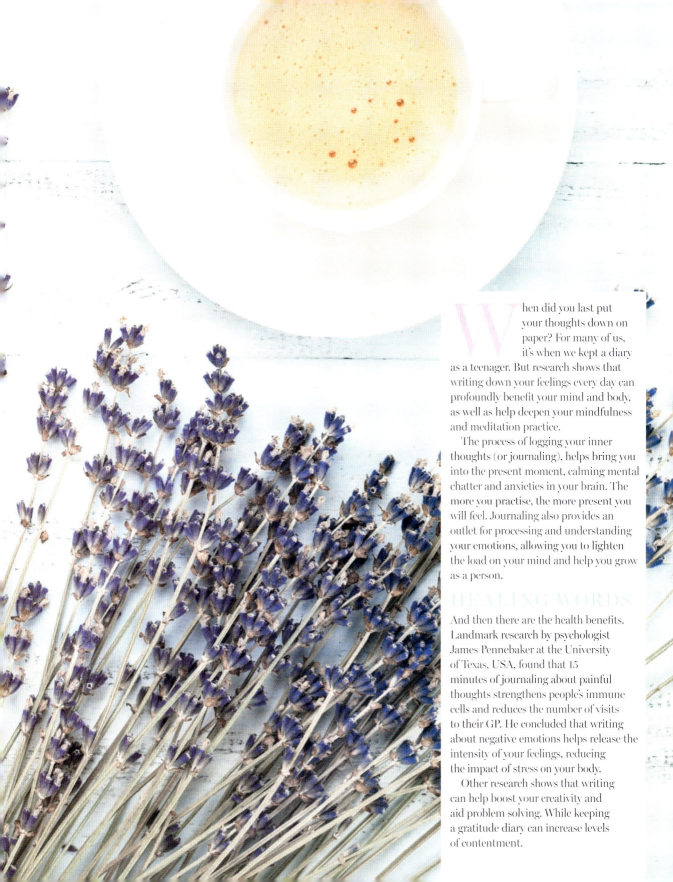

When did you last put your thoughts down on paper? For many of us, it's when we kept a diary as a teenager. But research shows that writing down your feelings every day can profoundly benefit your mind and body, as well as help deepen your mindfulness and meditation practice.

The process of logging your inner thoughts (or journaling), helps bring you into the present moment, calming mental chatter and anxieties in your brain. The more you practise, the more present you will feel. Journaling also provides an outlet for processing and understanding your emotions, allowing you to lighten the load on your mind and help you grow as a person.

HEALING WORDS

And then there are the health benefits. Landmark research by psychologist James Pennebaker at the University of Texas, USA, found that 15 minutes of journaling about painful thoughts strengthens people's immune cells and reduces the number of visits to their GP. He concluded that writing about negative emotions helps release the intensity of your feelings, reducing the impact of stress on your body.

Other research shows that writing can help boost your creativity and aid problem solving. While keeping a gratitude diary can increase levels of contentment.

HOW TO START

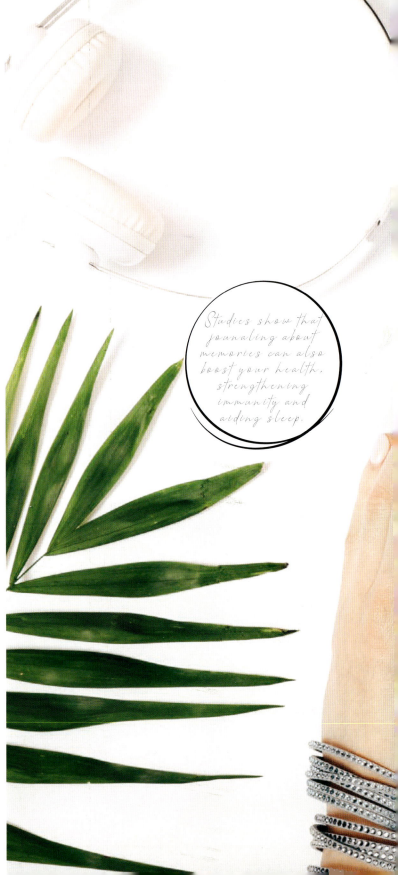

● Start small. Buy a pretty notebook you love to keep close.

● Keep it next to your bed, so you see it when you wake up. Take time in the morning and in the evening to write in it. This starts and finishes your day well.

● Write down three things you're grateful for — big or small.

● There are no rules about what to write. Note down what comes up in your mind, anything that keeps your mind or soul busy. Stay honest to yourself.

● Write three things that happened to you today — a few words or whole paragraphs, positive or negative. It's a chance to let everything out and can throw up interesting insights.

● To aid your practice, try writing down your three mindful moments and acknowledge your progress (try the journal pages in this book).

● Notice common themes? Write them down for extra attention.

● Set aside a regular time for your journal — first thing in the morning, last thing at night or your favourite quiet time of day.

Studies show that journaling about memories can also boost your health, strengthening immunity and aiding sleep.

'WHY I JOURNAL'

VERONIEK VERMEULEN IS FOUNDER OF THE SILATHA MEDITATION JOURNAL (SILATHA.COM)

'I ALWAYS KNEW ABOUT THE MANY BENEFITS OF JOURNALING, BUT HAD NEVER FELT A REAL URGE TO TRY IT BEFORE. I STARTED WITH A SMALL BOOKLET NEXT TO MY BED TO WRITE DOWN MY GRATITUDE. THEN, WHEN I STARTED MEDITATING, I FELT AN URGE TO EXPRESS MY FEELINGS, NOTING DOWN WHAT HAPPENED DURING THE MEDITATIONS. THIS HELPED ME PROCESS THE EXERCISES MORE DEEPLY, AND HELP MY LEARNING BECOME MORE ENGRAINED. WE THEN DEVELOPED THE SILATHA JOURNAL. IT GIVES ME IDEAS AND TIPS, WHILE ALSO OFFERING ENOUGH SPACE TO WRITE FREELY.

'JOURNALING GIVES YOU A FREEDOM – YOU CAN WRITE ABOUT ANYTHING AND IT TAKES YOU FURTHER ON YOUR JOURNEY. WRITING DOWN YOUR THOUGHTS AND FEELINGS GIVES YOU CLARITY AND PERSPECTIVE, HELPING YOU UNDERSTAND YOURSELF BETTER. IN TURN, YOUR THOUGHTS BECOME MORE PROFOUND. IT HELPS YOU GROW AND PROVIDES DIRECTION. COMBINING A MEDITATION PRACTICE WITH JOURNALING REALLY SUPPORTS YOUR WELLBEING!'

Once you've learnt the basics, you can try 'stream of consciousness' journaling. Simply write anything that comes into your head without editing or censoring. It unclutters your mind and boosts creativity.

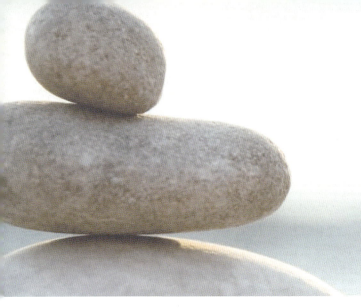

Can't access any natural space? Try visualising a beautiful place of nature you've visited in the past.

GET BACK TO NATURE

Want a shortcut to mindfulness? It's time to get outdoors

Even if you're new to mindfulness, you've probably already witnessed the feeling of inner calm when you've walked in the countryside or soaked up the sunshine. The sound of falling rain, the feeling of fresh air filling your lungs, the joyfulness of watching skipping lambs – these natural pleasures connect your true, inner self to the power of the universe. Put simply, spending time in nature is a direct line to instant calm.

Many ancient philosophies and healing systems have their roots in the natural world, from the totems of the Native American Indians to the meditations of Zen Buddhism. And now, modern science is proving there was good reason. Study after study confirm that spending time in nature helps boost mood, reduce clinical depression, lower blood pressure and boost creativity. The biggest benefits of all come from combining nature with exercise – whether it's hiking in the mountains or doing yoga in your garden. And research shows that meditation is easier outdoors too – instead of struggling with distractions, we're drawn to the aliveness of the present moment, achieving the state of 'samadhi' or effortless attention.

TRY THIS NATURE MEDITATION FROM MEDITATION MASTER NEIL SELIGMAN

Find a natural space that inspires you – it could be a lake or forest or simply your local park or garden.

1 Find a comfortable posture and take a few minutes to arrive and settle your breath into awareness.

2 Meet the natural world with the simplicity of your breath. Take five breaths.

3 Look around slowly, paying attention to anything that arouses your curiosity.

4 What can you see that is alive? Take five breaths here.

5 What can you hear that is alive? Take five breaths here.

6 What can you smell that is alive? Take five breaths here.

7 What do you feel that is alive? Take five breaths here.

8 Continue breathing and notice how you're connected to this place.

9 Allow the division between you and what you're seeing to slip away.

10 Become part of the scene, breathing in and out of the life that surrounds you.

11 Listen.

12 Breathe.

13 Listen.

14 Return to wakefulness.

Day 4

START A JOURNAL TONIGHT. WRITE ABOUT YOUR DAY AND HOW YOU FELT ABOUT WHAT HAPPENED. EVEN IF IT'S JUST A FEW LINES, THIS IS A GOOD EXERCISE IN BECOMING AWARE OF YOUR EMOTIONS AND BEGINNING TO VIEW THEM WITHOUT JUDGEMENT.

HOW I FELT

TODAY'S MINDFUL MOMENTS

Day 5

FIND A QUIET SPACE. IN THEORY, YOU CAN MEDITATE ANYWHERE, BUT IT'S GREAT TO HAVE A GO-TO SPOT YOU CAN RETREAT TO REGULARLY. IT DOESN'T HAVE TO BE A DEDICATED MEDITATION ROOM. PERHAPS THERE'S A COMFORTABLE SPOT IN YOUR BEDROOM OR A CORNER IN YOUR LIVING ROOM WHERE YOU CAN PLACE A CUSHION. IT MAY EVEN BE UNDER A TREE IN YOUR LOCAL PARK. (SEE P48 FOR MORE ADVICE.)

HOW I FELT

TODAY'S MINDFUL MOMENTS

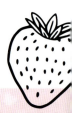

Day 6

LISTEN WELL. WE'RE OFTEN SO FOCUSED ON OUR PART IN A CONVERSATION, WE DON'T TRULY LISTEN TO THE OTHER PERSON. PRACTISE MINDFUL LISTENING. PAY ATTENTION TO THE OTHER PERSON'S WORDS, TONE OF VOICE, FACIAL EXPRESSIONS AND HAND GESTURES. NOTICE HOW OFTEN YOU THINK ABOUT YOUR RESPONSE TO WHAT THEY'RE SAYING. EVERY TIME THOSE THOUGHTS COME UP, ALLOW THEM TO SLIP AWAY AND GO BACK TO WHAT THAT PERSON IS SAYING.

HOW I FELT

TODAY'S MINDFUL MOMENTS

'You are the sky.
Everything else is
just weather'

PEMA CHODRON

MINDFUL MEDITATION

The art of meditation is a key way to develop greater mindfulness, and it brings with it a wealth of extra benefits for mind and body. In this section, you'll discover the science behind the ancient practice and learn how it can change the way your brain works for the better. Find out everything you need to get started and try some basic beginner's meditation exercises – it's easier than you think! Then, develop your practice with more advanced techniques, including a loving kindness meditation that will help bring happiness to yourself and those around you.

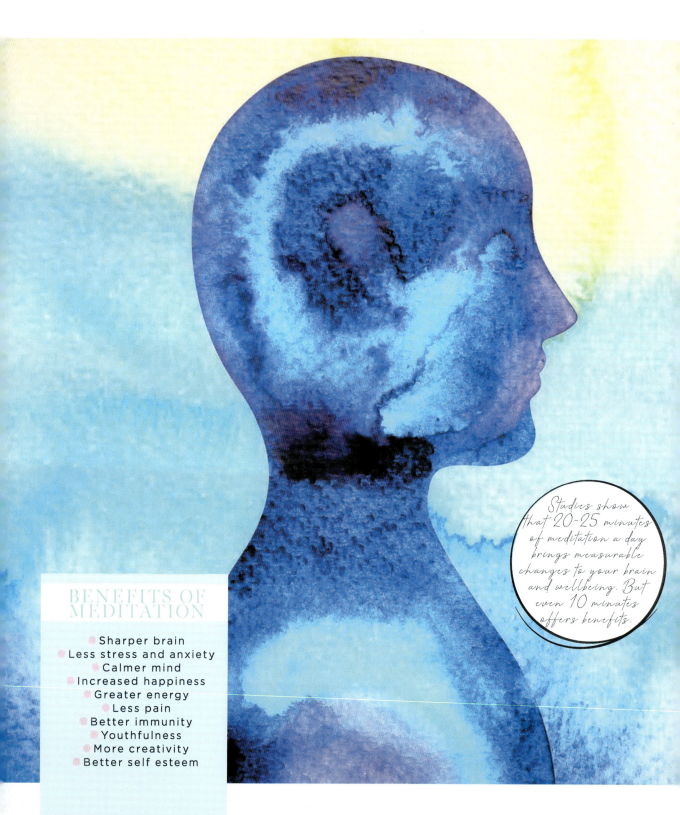

BENEFITS OF MEDITATION

* Sharper brain
* Less stress and anxiety
* Calmer mind
* Increased happiness
* Greater energy
* Less pain
* Better immunity
* Youthfulness
* More creativity
* Better self esteem

Studies show that 20-25 minutes of meditation a day brings measurable changes to your brain and wellbeing. But even 10 minutes offers benefits.

WHAT IS MEDITATION?

Now you've experienced what mindfulness feels like, here's how to deepen your practice

Meditation may sound mysterious but it's simply a more formal way to develop your mindfulness. Having a regular meditation practice trains your mind to become aware and be present without judgement or attachment. It can help bring structure to your mindfulness journey and allow you to develop and progress.

You don't need any special skills, religious belief or spirituality to meditate. You simply need to set aside some time, ideally every day, for a meditation session. Even 10 minutes is good to begin with.

FROM RELIGION TO SCIENCE

In the East, meditation has been used as a spiritual practice for thousands of years. Take Buddhist meditation for example. In the West, it's largely been used as a relaxation therapy. But recently, science has confirmed that meditation triggers physical changes in the brain that confer many more benefits for mental and physical health. And the more you practise, the more your brain changes – a process that is called neuroplasticity.

BRAIN BENEFITS

By studying electrical activity in the brain during meditation, neuroscientists discovered the practice changes the way our brains process fear. This leads to a reduction in stress and anxiety which also improves your immunity and resistance to infection and sickness. It may even slow down the ageing process.

Meditation develops areas of the brain associated with positive emotions and empathy, helping to reduce depression and enhance your relationships with others. And it activates the pre-frontal cortex of your brain, helping you think more clearly and make more measured decisions. Meanwhile, the deep relaxation that meditation brings can help restore and energise both your body and mind, and improve your sleep.

FIND YOUR PRACTICE

There are many methods of meditation practice but all combine two key elements: focusing the attention (for example on an object, your breath or a mantra) and mindful awareness without judgement.

Methods range from the basic body scan exercise (p52) and breath awareness (p30) to counting your breath, chanting and gazing at an object such as a flame (p58). Try to experiment with a few methods to begin with to find the one that suits you best.

LET'S GET STARTED

Meditation is easier than you think. Just follow these basic steps

A t it's most fundamental, meditation is one of the simplest ways to deeply relax you'll find. All you need to meditate is yourself and a quiet space. And once you've mastered the basics, it's something you'll be able to draw on in daily life wherever and whenever you need.

BEFORE YOU START

Choose a quiet place where you won't be disturbed. Somewhere clear and uncluttered will help clear your mind. You don't need any special clothes, just something loose and comfortable. Make sure the room or space is a comfortable temperature – too cold and it will distract you, too warm and you may find yourself drifting off to sleep. Keep a shawl handy in case you feel chilled and, ideally, have a window you can open if it gets too warm.

HOW TO SIT

To meditate effectively, you need to be able to sit comfortably for the duration of your practice – it's difficult to relax your mind if your body is in pain. Sitting, rather than lying down to meditate allows you to be relaxed yet alert. But don't worry if you're not flexible enough to sit cross-legged on the ground – there's no right or wrong way to sit for meditation. Many people choose to sit in a straight-backed chair. Here are some tips:

Sit up straight but relaxed to allow energy to circulate and your breath to be full.

EASY CROSS-LEGGED POSE

● Sit with your legs crossed loosely in front of you.
● If your back curves or your knees are higher than your hips, sit on a cushion or bolster to bring you into alignment and keep you grounded.
● Sit up straight but relaxed. Keep your chin parallel to the ground, gently tucked in.
● Draw your shoulders down your back to let any tension melt away and create space to breathe.

In Eastern traditions, it's thought the cross-legged pose enhances inward focus and the flow of prana (energy) around your body without it leaking away.

SITTING ON A CHAIR

● Choose a straight-backed chair. Sit upright with your back and buttocks away from the back of the chair. Place your hands on your knees. Keep your feet flat on the floor to ground you. If your knees are higher than your pelvis, place a folded blanket under your buttocks.
● Sit up straight but relaxed — imagine your head is being pulled gently upwards. Keep your chin tucked in slightly. Relax your shoulders.

KNEELING ON YOUR HEELS

● If you want to sit on the floor, you might prefer to sit on your heels instead of cross-legged. It's a pose used in Zen meditation.
● Kneel with your knees and feet together, buttocks on your heels.
● If it's uncomfortable to sit on your heels, place a cushion or rolled up blanket between your buttocks and heels.
● Keep the front of your shins on the ground.

Day 7

TAKE A FIVE-MINUTE MINDFUL WALK. YOU CAN FIT THIS IN ANY TIME, WHETHER IT'S PART OF YOUR REGULAR WEEKEND STROLL IN THE PARK OR YOUR WALK TO THE STATION ON THE WAY TO WORK. FOR FIVE MINUTES (YOU CAN TIME YOURSELF WITH YOUR PHONE), TAKE OUT YOUR EARPHONES, LOOK AROUND YOU AND BE FULLY PRESENT. NOTICE THE SOUNDS — EVERYTHING FROM BIRDSONG TO TRAFFIC NOISE AND PEOPLE TALKING. PAY ATTENTION TO SMELLS — COFFEE AS YOU PASS AN OPEN WINDOW AND ROTTING LEAVES, FOR EXAMPLE — AND TO THE FEELING OF THE BREEZE AGAINST YOUR SKIN, OR LIGHT RAIN FALLING AGAINST YOUR FACE. TRY TO BRING YOUR ATTENTION TO WHAT'S GOING ON AROUND YOU, LETTING THOUGHTS COME AND GO LIKE CLOUDS.

HOW I FELT

TODAY'S MINDFUL MOMENTS

Day 8

CREATE A MINDFUL MORNING ROUTINE. IT HELPS SET THE TONE FOR A CALMER DAY AHEAD. YOU DON'T HAVE TO DO ANYTHING SPECIAL — IT'S MORE ABOUT CREATING SPACE BEFORE YOU LET THE DAY IN. PERHAPS YOU'LL TAKE 10 MINUTES TO SIP HOT WATER AND LEMON BY THE WINDOW AS THE SUN RISES, DO A FEW SUN SALUTATIONS OR READ A QUOTE FROM AN INSPIRING BOOK. THIS MAY ALSO BECOME A GOOD TIME FOR YOUR MEDITATION. BUT FOR NOW, SIMPLY AIM TO START HAVING A SHORT MORNING RITUAL.

HOW I FELT

TODAY'S MINDFUL MOMENTS

Day 9

SIT STILL. FINDING THE RIGHT POSTURE IS CRUCIAL FOR MEDITATION SO GETTING USED TO SITTING IS GREAT PREPARATION. IDEALLY, SIT CROSS-LEGGED ON THE FLOOR, WITH A CUSHION TO SUPPORT YOUR BUM. OR YOU COULD SIT ON A CHAIR, FEET FLAT ON THE FLOOR, BUT MAKE SURE YOU DON'T SLUMP — YOUR SPINE SHOULD BE RELAXED BUT STRAIGHT, LEGS UNCROSSED, HANDS IN YOUR LAP. EXPERIMENT WITH GETTING THE RIGHT POSITION AND START BY JUST SITTING QUIETLY FOR TWO MINUTES.

HOW I FELT

_____

_____

_____

_____

TODAY'S MINDFUL MOMENTS

_____

_____

_____

_____

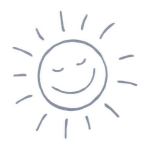

PREPARE TO PRACTISE

It's a lot easier than you think to create space in your day for mindfulness. Here's how…

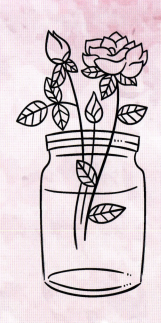

When you're juggling a busy life, finding time to meditate can seem an impossible task. But, it needn't be. 'Your breath and body will always be ready and available to lead you into present moment awareness,' says mindfulness advocate Neil Seligman, author of *100 Mindfulness Meditations* (Conscious House, £12.99). Follow his tips to get out of your head and into a more mindful way of being.

1. GO SHOPPING

You don't need to spend a lot of money, but investing in some tools for your practice will help support you on your mindfulness journey, says Seligman. A meditation cushion can be helpful, and a timer with an alarm allows you to relax into the experience without worrying about being late for your next commitment. And buy a beautiful notepad to use as a mindfulness journal. Seligman suggests one with an inspiring cover and blank pages. The blank pages will challenge you to be creative as you write your journal, so if you feel the urge, doodle or draw something alongside your notes.

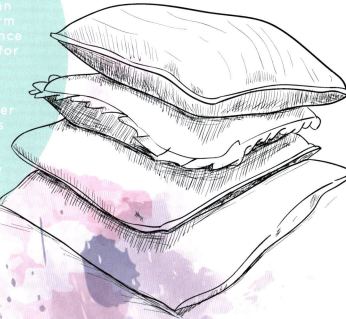

2 START SMALL

Don't set yourself up for failure. Start with a five-minute practice and gradually build up to 20 minutes. But it's important to make mindfulness work for you. Be flexible and accept that some days you won't be able to fit in much practice, but at other times you'll be able to dedicate more time to meditate. Most of all, observe how your mind and body respond to different periods of meditation and find the right duration for your lifestyle.

3 CREATE A RITUAL

Following the same sequence each time you practise will help you tune in more quickly. 'For me, that means picking up my cushion, placing it in front of the window, setting up my timer and placing my mindfulness journal, pen and cup of chamomile tea at my side,' says Seligman. 'I then take my seat and begin my practice.' You can enhance the impact of your ritual further by bringing present moment awareness to each of these acts of simple preparation. They become part of the practice itself.

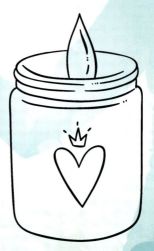

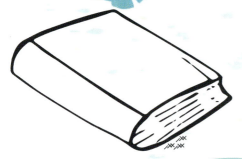

SUPPORT YOUR PRACTICE

Need extra guidance for your mindful journey? Try a guided meditation or mindfulness app. Here are a few suggestions:
Headspace: free download gives you 10 days of guided meditations (headspace.com).
Calm: free download gives voice-led meditations including a seven-day beginner's programme (calm.com).
Aura: free download for daily three-minute meditations and calming sounds (aurahealth.io).

4. MIX IT UP

Different mindfulness practices develop different skills and a varied practice keeps you interested. 'One day I use an open-monitoring practice to simply notice what is arising within me,' says Seligman. 'On another I take a single focus, such as my breath or a flame. Sometimes I focus on a person I love and absorb the feelings of support and compassion that arise as I visualise them with me.'

5 EMBRACE DISTRACTIONS

Rather than fight a wandering mind, noisy neighbour or aching back, work with it and use it as an opportunity to teach yourself awareness and focus. Seligman has learnt to turn his Labrador's attentions into a mindful meditation in itself. 'I close my eyes, he nuzzles my ears. I centre myself, he licks my face. I ignore him, he sits squarely on my lap,' he recounts. 'Sometimes, he gives up his nuzzling and sits quietly at my side. Other times I acquiesce, we play together and I try to be fully present with him. Ty has taught me that an authentic mindfulness practice cannot be overly rigid and must include space for the spontaneous and the unexpected.'

GO EASY

There will be days or weeks when your mindfulness practice goes on the back burner. Self-acceptance is vital for long-term success. 'Without forgiveness it may be impossible to find your way back,' says Seligman. 'So, each time you miss a practice, forgive yourself as immediately and completely as you can. Try not to let guilty feelings of missing practice keep you away from the rich possibility of your next meditation.'

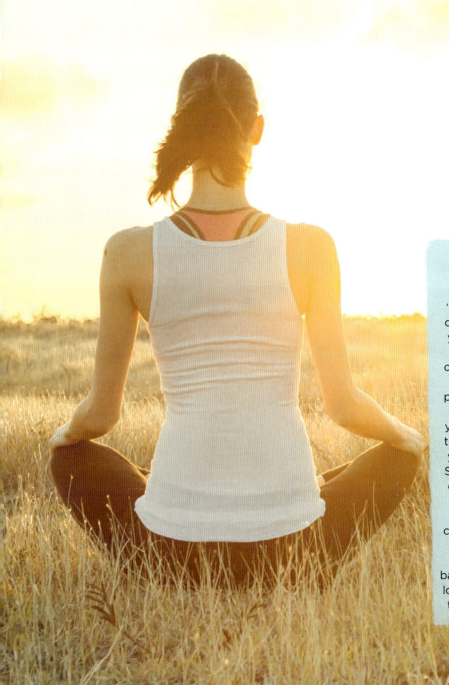

'IT WORKS FOR ME'

Veroniek Vermeulen

Wellpreneur

'Meditation is the moment of the day that is purely for you. It gives you so much peace and balance for the rest of the day. I'm convinced that if the whole world meditated, it would be a better place for all of us, as it makes you connect to the energy around you. When you feel connected to the world, you feel more love and you give more love and warmth. So it's not only a beautiful way to create inner peace and a feeling of fulfilment, it also supports your surroundings with more calm and peace. And it helps give perspective. After doing a meditation series, I look back – sometimes I've developed a lot, sometimes I realise I had been there all along without noticing.'

BODY SCAN
MEDITATION

Ready to get started? This relaxing exercise is one of the foundations of mindfulness practice

The body scan is a mindfulness meditation that expands your sense of awareness through your physical body. By shifting your attention slowly from one area of your body to another and tuning in to the physical sensations of each body part, you learn to bring your attention to the here and now and to anchor your mind in the present moment.

WHAT TO EXPECT

As you move from one body part to the next, you'll start to notice sensations, such as stiffness, tension or your heartbeat. Sometimes these feelings may be intense, sometimes they will be barely perceptible. Scientific research shows that doing a body scan meditation can help reduce physical pain and reduce stress.

You may also notice emotional feelings as you tune into a body part. This is because we all hold experiences and memories in our body. It's totally normal; simply acknowledge your feelings without dwelling on them or trying to change anything.

This exercise should be nurturing, so approach your body with a kind, gentle curiosity, without any judgement or expectation. Don't become impatient or frustrated if you lose focus, the more you practise, the longer you'll be able to sustain your attention.

Try doing the body scan every day for a week to get accustomed to it. Allow at least half a minute for each body part. Ideally, spend 30-45 minutes in total.

1 Get into a comfortable position, whatever that may be – on a yoga mat or rug. Take a moment to let your mind settle and your heart slow down. Gradually bring your attention to your breath and notice how your body is responding.

Breathe in through your nose and imagine your breath travelling through your body to and out of the body part you're focusing on. Then reverse this as you breathe in.

2 When ready, transfer your attention to the toes of your left foot. Focus on each toe in turn, noticing any sensations. Is there warmth, coldness or tingling? Acknowledge any thoughts that arise, simply returning your attention to your toes. Use your breath to guide you, taking it right down to the bottom of your foot on the inhale and back up it on the exhale. Next, rest your attention on the sole of your left foot, becoming aware of any sensation you feel here. Then, move your focus to the top of your foot and your ankle.

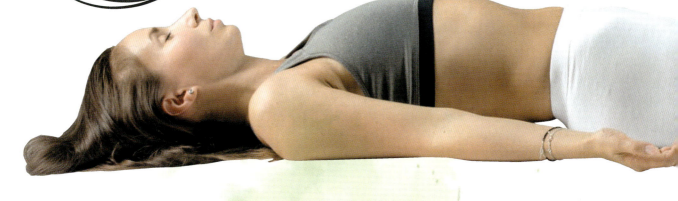

7 Gently take your attention to your left arm - first the fingertips of your left hand and moving up to your left shoulder via your lower arm, elbow and upper arm. Repeat the pattern on your right arm.

6 Next, move your attention to your chest and upper back, focusing your awareness on the rise and fall of your rib cage as you breathe. Be aware of your lungs and heart too.

8 Now move your attention to your neck and throat, and then your face. Let go of any tension in your jaw and cheeks and notice the sensation of your tongue relaxing against the roof of your mouth and your lips touching together.

3 After a deep inhale, move your attention to your left calf and shin. As you breathe, sense not just your muscles and skin but deep into your bones. Continue moving in this way to incorporate more and more of your body, travelling to your left knee, thigh and hip, all the time allowing yourself to rest in the present.

4 After pausing for a moment at your left hip, take your attention to your right leg, focusing first on your toes, and progressing to the sole, heel and top of your right foot, then to your calf, shin, knee, thigh and hip.

5 Coming from your right hip, let your attention fall onto your pelvic area – your groin and buttocks - letting your attention expand into the area as you inhale, softening, and then releasing on an exhale. Once you're ready, move your focus to your lower torso, feeling your lower back sink into the floor. Breathe into the area before letting go on an exhale and moving onto your abdomen. Be aware of it moving as you breathe.

9 Become aware of your eyes and eyelids, letting them soften into your face. Then progress to your forehead, ears, and the back and top of your head, breathing into each area and experiencing whatever is present for you.

10 Once you've scanned every body part, focus your attention on your body as a whole, breathing in to your entire body. Feel it open and expand, soften and release. Feel yourself present and fully awake in this moment.

11 When you're ready to come out of the body scan, take a couple of deep breaths and become aware of the ground beneath you. Gently wriggle your fingers and toes and stretch your body, before slowly opening your eyes and coming back to sitting. If you like, you can jot down your experiences in a journal, to see how they develop and change over repeated practice.

ENGAGE YOUR
SENSES

Struggle to empty your mind of thoughts? Learn how to focus your mind with this easy exercise

If you've never meditated before or struggle to calm your mental chatter, one of the easiest ways to start is to meditate on an object. In most Eastern traditions a candle flame is used. But choosing an object that you can handle and observe in minute detail, engaging every sense, offers a perfect way to engage your senses and stay present. In his mindfulness-based stress reduction programme, Jon Kabat-Zinn suggests using a raisin. But you can apply the technique to any object. Here's how...

WHAT YOU NEED

Choose an object you can explore, smell and even taste, such as a piece of fruit or a flower. Find a quiet space where you won't be disturbed and turn off your phone.

1. Close your eyes and tune into your breath, allowing it to settle and deepen. When you're ready, pick up your chosen object, such as a peach, and look at it as if you're seeing it for the first time..

2. After a while, pick up the peach with gentle curiosity. Hold it in your hands, while continuing to observe it.

3. Notice how the peach feels against your skin and how it sits in your hands.

4. Focus on the temperature of the peach – does it feel warm or cool against your skin?

5. Now, focus on the texture of the peach – does it feel rough or smooth? Is the surface even or irregular? Is it damp or dry?

6. Move your attention to the colour of the peach. Is it evenly coloured or patterned? Turn it over in your hands. Are there variations or blemishes?

7. Bring the peach to your nose – does it have a fragrance? Inhale and savour its smell.

8. Slowly bring the peach to your mouth. Notice your reaction as you hold it to your lips.

9. Take a small bite and close your mouth. Not yet chewing, become aware of the sensations occurring in your mouth.

10. Slowly move the peach around your mouth with your tongue. What do you notice?

11. Now bite into the peach. What sensations do you feel? Slowly chew, noticing how the texture changes in your mouth.

12. What does the peach taste like? Sweet, salty, acidic? Notice the sensations it triggers in your mouth.

13. How does your mouth feel now it is empty? Can you feel a difference in your stomach?

14. Sit for a few moments, allowing your body to absorb the benefits. Then return to your day, taking with you some of the mindful stillness.

TIP: If your attention wanders or you find yourself wondering what you're doing, acknowledge the thoughts and perhaps say 'thinking'

MEDITATION EXERCISES

Take your practice further with these classic techniques

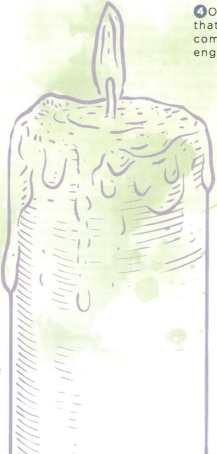

1 GAZING AT AN OBJECT

This meditation practice, called trataka, is said to purify the mind and improve concentration, enabling you to deepen your practice.

Why it works: By fixing your gaze on the object, you remove all distractions and your mind becomes still.

Benefits: Enhances focus, awareness and attention.

To start: Find a place where you won't be disturbed. Set a candle a few feet away from you, at eye level. Choose a sitting position and get comfortable. Set a timer for 10 minutes.

1 Close your eyes and spend a few moments connecting to your breath, settling into its natural rhythm.

2 Light the candle and sit back down in front it.

3 Gently gaze at the flame, focusing purely on its flickering presence and nothing else.

4 Observe any thoughts that arise, letting them come and go without engaging with them.

5 Breathe and connect with the flame, watching and feeling its movements as you breathe.

6 Feel the light of the candle flowing in and out of yourself as you breathe, fully absorbing yourself in the sensation.

7 When you're ready to finish, gently close your eyes, breathe into your belly and absorb your experiences.

SO HAM MEDITATION

This yogic practice uses a mantra to take you to a deeper level of focus.

Why it works: It uses the mantra 'so ham' which both reflects the sound of your breath and has a contemplative Sanskrit meaning 'I am that' ('so' = I am; 'ham' = that) pronounced as 'so hum'.

Benefits: It stimulates the throat chakra, cleansing your body, creating space in your mind and developing clarity and focus.

❶ Close your eyes and become aware of your breath. Take a few deep breaths and then let go.

❷ Tune in to the natural rhythm of your breath.

❸ Gradually, as you inhale, silently say 'so' and feel your breath draw in.

❹ As you exhale, say 'ham' and let go of any tension and thoughts.

❺ Follow this rhythmic pattern, fixing your attention on the sound of your breath as it says the mantra. If your mind drifts off, bring it back to your breath.

❻ Once you're ready to finish, bring your hands together in prayer position for a moment, to absorb the effects of the meditation.

To start: Find a comfortable position seated on a cushion or blanket, in a chair or against a wall. Sit up straight and with your chin slightly tucked in and neck long. Rest the backs of your hands on your thighs.

LOVING-KINDNESS MEDITATION

This Buddhist practice was designed to help monks cultivate selfless love and altruism. Beginning with self-compassion, the meditation broadens to embrace others with a wave of positive energy.

Why it works: It increases feelings of empathy, love and gratitude.

Benefits: It can help you feel more content with life, enrich your relationships, combat loneliness and make you feel connected to others.

Get started: Begin by getting into a comfortable sitting position and settling your breath. Let go of any thoughts.

1 Make a wish of loving kindness for yourself, silently repeating the following phrase. 'May I be filled with loving kindness.' Let your breath find a natural rhythm as you repeat the phrase, feeling the intention of the words as you say them. You might like to imagine yourself bathed in golden light or conjure up a memory of when you felt loved, then letting go of the memory and staying with the feeling. When you feel a warmth towards yourself arising, move onto the next step.

2 Bring to mind someone you care deeply about. Connect to your feelings for them and then make a wish of loving kindness for them. Address them directly by name '...may you be filled with loving kindness. May you enjoy happiness, peace and health.' Continue to breathe and repeat the phrases, feeling the sincerity as you say them. Sense your heart becoming open. You may like to visualise soft light travelling from your heart to your loved one. Continue to breathe and repeat the phrase..

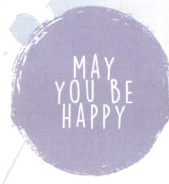

MAY YOU BE HAPPY

3 Make a wish of loving kindness to someone you have neutral feelings about. Perhaps a colleague at work or someone you haven't seen for a while. As you repeat the phrases, hold the person in your awareness offering your feelings for their wellbeing..

4 Now send loving kindness to someone you don't like or who has hurt or annoyed you. This will probably be challenging initially but the more you practise the easier it will become – once you've established self compassion, it's easier to feel it for others too. If negative feelings arise, simply acknowledge them and re-focus on their need for loving kindness.

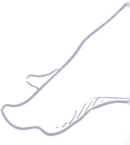

MAY I BE PEACEFUL

4 The final step of your meditation is to offer loving kindness to all beings and humanity in general.

5 To finish, gradually let your mind become still again. Spend a few moments absorbing your experience and the effects.

Begin with five minutes of loving-kindness meditation and build up your practice. Some experts recommend doing it for 15-20 minutes once or twice a day for several months.

BE FILLED WITH LOVING KINDNESS

Modern-day research has confirmed the value of this ancient practice. One study, published in the *Journal of Personality and Social Psychology* found that seven weeks of practice increased feelings of love, joy, contentment and gratitude, leading to a greater sense of purpose in life. And the benefits of loving-kindness meditation extend beyond happiness. Studies show it can relieve the symptoms of conditions such as back pain and migraine.

Day 10

BRING AWARENESS TO DOING THE WASHING UP. YES, EVEN A CHORE CAN BE A MINDFUL ACTIVITY! REALLY FOCUS ON WHAT YOU'RE DOING. NOTICE THE TEMPERATURE OF THE WATER ON YOUR HANDS, THE SENSATION OF BUBBLES AGAINST YOUR SKIN, THE FEEL OF THE PLATES AND CUTLERY AS YOU CLEAN THEM. CONCENTRATE ON GETTING THE DISHES CLEAN. WHEN OTHER THOUGHTS COME UP, BRING YOUR AWARENESS BACK TO THE WASHING UP.

HOW I FELT

TODAY'S MINDFUL MOMENTS

Day 11

WRITE A GRATITUDE LIST. THIS CAN HELP YOU APPRECIATE EVERYTHING IN YOUR LIFE AT THE MOMENT. THIS EVENING, WRITE DOWN EVERYTHING FOR WHICH YOU'VE BEEN GRATEFUL TODAY, FROM THAT COMFORTING AFTERNOON CUPPA TO THE TEXT YOU RECEIVED FROM A FRIEND. DO THIS DAILY AND YOU'LL START TO NOTICE THOSE SMALL, SIMPLE THINGS THAT MEAN SO MUCH.

HOW I FELT

TODAY'S MINDFUL MOMENTS

Day 12

PRACTISE MINDFULNESS OF SMELL. IT'S A SENSE WE CAN OFTEN FORGET ABOUT BUT IT GIVES US IMPORTANT INFORMATION AND CAN HELP US CONNECT WITH OUR EMOTIONS. LIGHT SOME INCENSE OR PUT ESSENTIAL OIL ONTO A TISSUE. CLOSE YOUR EYES, HOLD THE SCENT TO YOUR NOSE AND SNIFF. NOTICE ANY FEELINGS OR MEMORIES THAT RISE UP. SMELL MORE DEEPLY. AGAIN, NOTICE YOUR EMOTIONS WITHOUT JUDGING THEM — JUST ALLOW THEM TO COME AND GO. FULLY EXPERIENCE THE SCENT, PAYING ATTENTION TO ALL THE NOTES YOU CAN DETECT IN IT.

HOW I FELT

TODAY'S MINDFUL MOMENTS

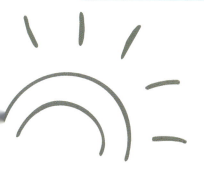

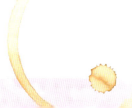

MUSICAL
HEALING

Does your mind keep
wandering when you're trying
to meditate? It's time to turn
up the music

When you start to practise mindful meditation, one of the most important moments comes when you realise that your attention has wandered. It's essential not to see this as a failure but as an opportunity to allow you to return to the focus of your practice. It shows that your awareness is growing.

This musical mindfulness exercise from mindfulness coach Neil Seligman will help you practise your focus.

HOW TO DO IT

Choose a piece of music and press play. Find a comfortable posture and bring your attention to your breath. Take a few moments to let yourself arrive and allow your breath to draw you gently into internal awareness. Allow your gaze to soften, and your eyes to close.

1 IMAGINE YOU COMPOSED THIS MUSIC; THAT IT FLOWED INTO THE WORLD DIRECTLY FROM YOUR HEART.

2 LISTEN WITH CLARITY AND ALLOW YOURSELF TO BE DRAWN INTO THE MELODY, THE RHYTHM, THE MOVEMENT AND THE EMOTION.

3 FEEL THE VIBRATION OF THE MUSIC IN EVERY CELL OF YOUR BODY.

4 WHAT EMOTIONS ARISE? PAY FULL ATTENTION TO ANY FEELINGS PRESENT AND NOTICE THEIR SUBTLE MOVEMENT THROUGH YOUR BODY.

5 IF YOUR MIND WANDERS FROM THE FOCUS OF THE MUSIC, BRING IT BACK PATIENTLY AND COMPASSIONATELY.

6 CONTINUE CONNECTING AND RECONNECTING WITH THE PIECE OF MUSIC.

7 IMAGINE THAT THE MUSIC IS FLOWING OUT OF YOU NOW.

8 WHAT DO YOU SEE? WHAT DO YOU FEEL? WHAT DO YOU SENSE?

9 TAKE FIVE BREATHS HERE.

10 BREATHE AND FOLLOW THE MUSIC UNTIL IT ENDS.

11 RETURN TO WAKEFULNESS IN YOUR OWN WAY. RECORD YOUR EXPERIENCE OF WHAT YOU SAW, FELT AND SENSED. IF PRACTISING WITH OTHERS, TAKE TURNS SHARING YOUR DISCOVERIES.

If you pick a favourite track, try to listen as if you're hearing it for the first time.

'Many people are alive but
don't touch the miracle
of being alive'

THICH NHAT HANH

EVERYDAY
MINDFULNESS

Now you've learnt the basics of mindfulness, it's time to apply your new knowledge to everyday life. Whether you want to be a calm commuter, beat office stress or tame the chaos of family life, mindfulness can help and the following pages will show you how. Try the simple daily exercises, learn how eating mindfully can help you lose weight and glean handy tips to help you keep your cool when the pace of life heats up.

ON THE MOVE

Now you've learnt the basics, you can apply mindfulness to your daily life – and your commute to work is the perfect opportunity

Does your journey to and from work drive you crazy? Do you get home from a day in the city feeling drained of energy? Do you rush though daily life barely noticing the changing seasons or your neighbours' attempts to strike up a conversation?

If life is passing you by in a blur of stress and fatigue, adding some simple mindfulness techniques into your daily life when you're out and about, can bring calm to the chaos and turn your mood around.

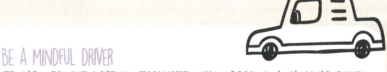

BE A MINDFUL DRIVER

IT'S EASY TO GET LOST IN THOUGHTS WHEN DRIVING A FAMILIAR ROUTE SO TRY THIS EXERCISE FOR A FEW MINUTES. TURN THE RADIO OFF AND NOTE THE SILENCE. NOW BRING YOUR ATTENTION TO YOUR DRIVING. NOTICE YOUR HANDS ON THE WHEEL AND WHAT IT FEELS LIKE. NOTICE YOUR FEET IN CONTACT WITH THE PEDALS AND YOUR BOTTOM ON THE SEAT. NOW BRING YOUR ATTENTION TO THE REST OF YOUR BODY. NOTICE IF YOUR SHOULDERS ARE TIGHT OR YOUR BACK HUNCHED. TAKE A FEW DEEP BREATHS AND RELEASE ANY TENSION. THEN NOTICE YOUR SURROUNDINGS, THE NEARBY CARS AND VIEW IN FRONT OF YOU. IF YOUR MIND WANDERS, GENTLY BRING YOUR FOCUS BACK.

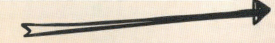

Switch your thinking

When your blood pressure is rising over yet another delay, it's time to shift your focus. Accept the fact there's nothing you can do about the situation and, instead, use the time as a chance to check in with yourself. Focus on your breathing and scan your body and mind – how are they feeling? Take a few deep breaths, exhaling any tension and notice the changes in how you're feeling. If you're sitting down and have five or 10 minutes, try the breath awareness exercise (p30).

GROUND YOURSELF

IF IMPATIENCE IS RISING AS YOU WAIT IN A QUEUE FOR THE BUS OR A CASH POINT, TAKE YOUR ATTENTION DOWN TO YOUR FEET. FEEL THE CONTACT BETWEEN THE SOLES OF YOUR FEET AND THE GROUND. TAKE YOUR BREATH FROM THE BASE OF YOUR SPINE, DOWN BOTH LEGS AND OUT THROUGH YOUR FEET INTO THE GROUND BELOW. NOTICE HOW THIS GROUNDING EXERCISE MAKES YOU FEEL

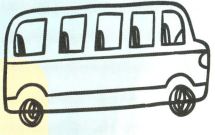

Be a kinder commuter

Feeling inner rage with that slow driver or the passenger who's elbowed you out of a seat? Try practising some loving kindness (p60). When negative thoughts start to simmer, take a deep breath and let them go. Send compassion to other commuters and try some random acts of kindness such as offering someone a seat. Creating mindful connections with your fellow travellers will turn your journeys into a more enjoyable experience.

Smile inside

Even if you're feeling grumpy, practising smiling on the inside will help you feel better. Simply imagine you're smiling. How does your face feel? How does your heart feel? How does the space around you feel? Remember, your experience of the present is not fixed but is dependent on your relationship with it.

LOOK UP

IT'S TEMPTING TO BLOT OUT YOUR JOURNEY BY SCROLLING ON YOUR SMARTPHONE. BUT TODAY, TRY PUTTING YOUR PHONE AWAY AND TAKE TIME TO OBSERVE YOUR SURROUNDINGS. NOTICE THE FACES OF PEOPLE IN YOUR CARRIAGE, THE DETAILS OF HOUSES OR OTHER BUILDINGS YOU'RE PASSING, THE CLOUDS IN THE SKY OR THE SETTING SUN. YOU'LL BE SURPRISED AT WHAT YOU'VE BEEN MISSING!

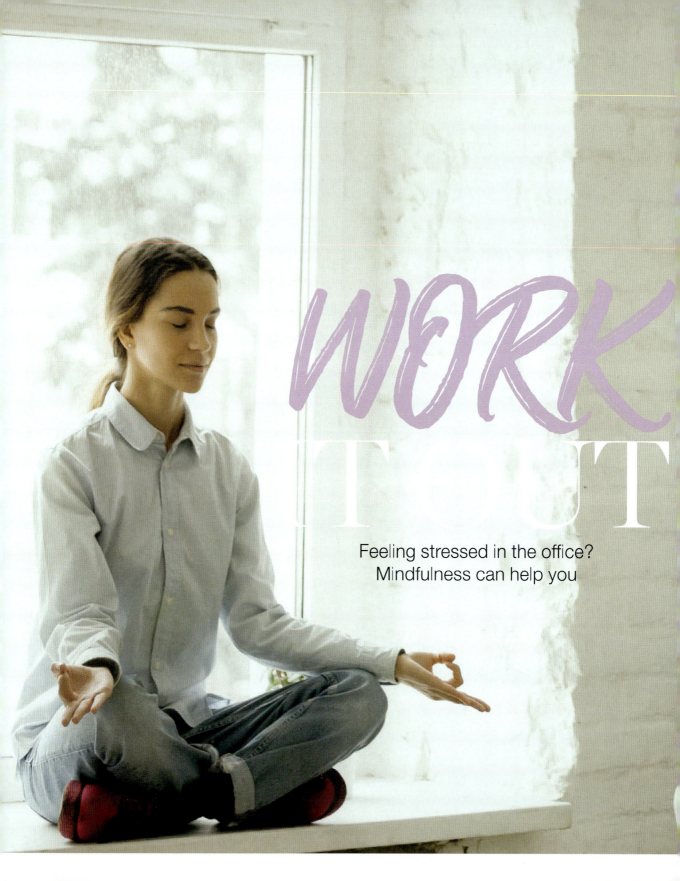

WORK OUT

Feeling stressed in the office?
Mindfulness can help you

It's 5 o'clock on a Friday, you're itching to escape for the weekend but there's a pile of work in front of you and the boss has just handed you an urgent deadline. Take a deep breath – new research shows that applying the principles of mindfulness to your working day can stop stress in its tracks. And you don't even need to leave your desk – though that might be a good idea...

Try doing these exercises from mindfulness instructor Anna Black, author of *Mindfulness @ Work* (Cico Books, £12.99) whenever the pressure starts to build.

TIP: Practising mindfulness at work will mean you're better able to problem-solve when issues do arise.

EMBRACE THE GOOD

Have you noticed you're more likely to remember a negative or annoying situation at work than a normal experience? As humans we're programmed to be vigilant to threats so our body/mind doesn't store positive experiences in the same way. If you can take note of a positive experience as it happens, you can 'bank' it in your body memory.

✣ Notice any good experiences today. It could be a smile from a colleague, a blast of fresh air at lunchtime or a quick chat at the water cooler - anything that makes you feel good.

✣ Pay attention to this experience as it happens and allow yourself to feel it. What sensations do you notice? Where are they? What do they feel like? What thoughts and emotions are you aware of?

✣ You may be surprised to find there are more pleasant experiences in your day than you thought. By noticing them, you're acknowledging a more balanced view of your life and storing them in your body's emotional memory.

✣ Try writing down your experience and reflect on what has happened. Are there particular tasks or people you respond to positively?

1

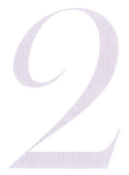

2 TAKE A MINDFUL MOMENT

Calm down in 20 seconds with The Mindful Minute, a simple calming meditation you can do at your desk.

✣ When you need to de-stress, settle your attention on your breath and count each in- and out-breath, from one up to the number of breaths you counted earlier. This is your mindful minute. Do this every so often throughout the day and you'll increase your minutes of present-moment awareness with all the mental and physical benefits this brings.

✣ While you're feeling stressed, count the number of breaths you take in a minute.

'IT WORKS FOR ME'
Emma Brown
Copywriter, London

'When I don't meditate, my working day is usually spent hunched over a computer, my muscles tense and my breathing becomes shallow. My mind races and I barely eat or drink. All I want to do at the end of the day is collapse in front of the TV. If I meditate before the day begins, it's a different experience. I'm present in my body and there's space to think more creatively. Deadlines are more manageable and I feel more satisfied at the end of the day. I also have more energy in the evening. Even just checking in throughout the day with mindful breathing or a quick body scan helps me come back to the present and choose more consciously how I spend my time.'

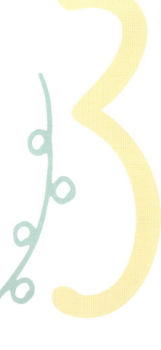

SIT TALL

Your neck and shoulders are often the first areas of your body to tense and stiffen when you're stressed. By paying attention to your posture when you're siting at your desk or in a meeting you'll notice your patterns and stop tension in its tracks. It's only when you bring something into awareness that you have the capacity to do it differently. Your external posture often reflects the internal state of your mind. Notice the connection between your mind and body.

✣ Plant your feet on the floor.

✣ Imagine a thread running all the way up your spine, along the back of your neck and out through the crown of your head.

✣ Give the thread a gentle tug so your spine lengthens, the crown of your head lifts to the ceiling and your chin becomes tucked in.

✣ You should now be sitting tall, the lower half of your body grounded and connected to the earth with your torso rising up. Realising how your posture reflects your state of mind allows you to make adjustments, says Black.

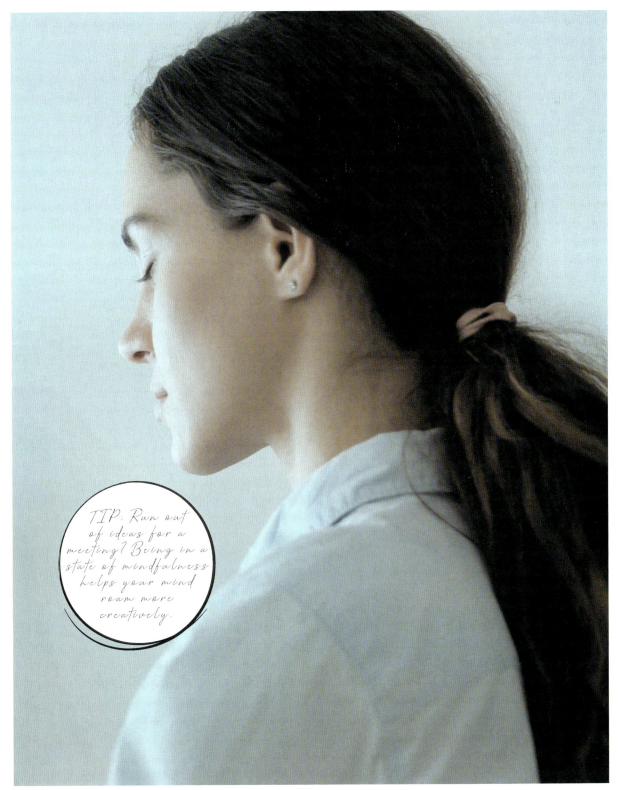

TIP: Run out of ideas for a meeting? Being in a state of mindfulness helps your mind roam more creatively.

AND BREATHE

Feeling wound up and impatient? Here's how to stay calm…

Ever stormed out of a shop when you've been stuck in a queue? Or found yourself cursing in a traffic jam? If so, then you're part of a modern phenomenon – impatience. Research shows most of us these days reach boiling point after waiting for a mere two and a half minutes!

Of course, it's natural to feel wound up by certain elements of life. According to stress experts, we feel at our most stressed when we have no control over something, whether it's a traffic jam or automated voice on the other end of the line. And being short of time – another feature of our modern lives – makes waiting all the more frustrating.

Ultimately, bursting with impatience usually achieves little and harms nobody but you. If you're constantly getting impatient, the resulting stress can lead to depression, unhealthy coping behaviours, such as heavy drinking, or even physical conditions including headaches and IBS. Here's how to stay calm when you start to lose your cool.

HOW IMPATIENT ARE YOU?

Tick any of the following that apply.

1. I GET IRRITATED WHEN I CAN'T UNDERSTAND SOMETHING.

2. I NEVER READ INSTRUCTION MANUALS.

3. I GET FRUSTRATED WHEN I'M TRYING TO EXPLAIN SOMETHING TO SOMEONE AND THEY'RE SLOW TO GRASP IT.

4. I FEEL ANNOYED IF I HAVE TO WAIT FOR SOMETHING FOR MORE THAN A FEW MINUTES.

5. I'M MORE LIKELY TO LEAVE A LONG QUEUE THAN WAIT TILL I GET TO THE FRONT.

6. I OFTEN PUT THE PHONE DOWN WHEN I'M PUT ON HOLD.

7. SLOW WIFI MAKES MY BLOOD BOIL AND SOMETIMES HAS ME IN TEARS.

ACCEPT: CAN YOU DO ANYTHING PRACTICAL ABOUT THE DELAYED TRAIN/LONG QUEUE/SLOW WIFI? IF YOU CAN SORT ALTERNATIVE ARRANGEMENTS DO SO. IF NOT, ACCEPT YOU ARE POWERLESS OVER THE SITUATION. STOP FIGHTING IT MENTALLY AND YOU'LL INSTANTLY FEEL LESS STRESSED.

DEFUSE: YOU MAY NOT BE ABLE TO CHANGE THE SITUATION BUT YOU CAN TAKE STEPS TO MAKE IT LESS STRESSFUL. FOR EXAMPLE, LET YOUR BOSS KNOW YOU'LL BE LATE IF YOU'RE WAITING FOR A DELAYED TRAIN OR ASK SOMEONE FOR HELP WITH INSTRUCTIONS YOU CAN'T UNDERSTAND.

CALM YOURSELF: BREATHING IS THE KEY TO KEEPING COOL. INHALE SLOWLY THROUGH YOUR NOSE AND RELEASE YOUR BREATH TO A COUNT OF FIVE. AFTER DOING THIS A FEW TIMES, YOU SHOULD FEEL SOOTHED. BE MINDFUL. OBSERVE YOUR IMPATIENT THOUGHTS AND SEE THEM FOR WHAT THEY ARE — JUST THOUGHTS.

RE-FRAME THE SITUATION: RATHER THAN THINKING OF IT AS A FRUSTRATION, LOOK AT THE TIME YOU'RE WAITING AS A CHANCE TO READ YOUR BOOK, MAKE A LIST OR LISTEN TO SOME MUSIC. IF YOUR ANNOYANCE IS WITH A PERSON, FOCUS ON THEM RATHER THAN YOURSELF — INSTEAD OF FEELING IRRITATED THAT THEY'RE NOT GRASPING WHAT YOU'RE EXPLAINING, THINK ABOUT HOW THEY'LL BENEFIT WHEN THEY DO UNDERSTAND.

BE A
MINDFUL EATER

Want to lose weight or eat more healthily? Eating mindfully is a key first step

Do you ever reach for the second half of your lunchtime sandwich only to realise you've already eaten it? Or guzzle a family-size bag of crisps while you're watching TV without even noticing what you've done? Thanks to busy lifestyles and an over-abundance of convenience food, for many of us, eating is an increasingly mindless activity. The result? Not only do we miss out on the sensual pleasure of eating but we're more likely to overeat, make poor food choices and struggle to maintain a healthy weight.

Mindful eating – paying attention to the experience of eating – is not only a useful way to practise and develop mindfulness (see page 56), it can also increase your enjoyment of food and turn around your health. Connecting to all your senses while you eat puts you in touch with your body's hunger signals, meaning you're more likely to stop eating when you're full, avoid mindless snacking or emotional eating and choose healthier foods.

In a study at North Carolina State University in the US, a group of people who followed a mindful eating programme for 15 weeks lost an average of 1.9kg. After six months, 75 per cent had not regained weight and some had lost more.

Try these mindful eating tips today and really start to enjoy your meals (see opposite page).

Buddhist monks chew each mouthful of food 30 times to aid their mindful awareness.

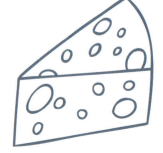

LISTEN TO YOUR BODY

Rather than automatically eating meals and snacks at set times, re-connect with your body's natural signals. Do you actually feel hungry or are you just eating out of habit? Respect your body's needs.

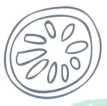

REFLECT AND APPRECIATE

As you eat, think about the food on your plate and where it has come from. Acknowledge your appreciation for the effort that has gone into producing it.

EAT MORE SLOWLY

Take smaller bites and chew your food slowly. Notice the texture and the flavour of the food you're eating, before you swallow. Health experts recommend chewing each mouthful up to 32 times for good digestion.

CUT THE CHAT

Socialising over a meal is one of life's simplest pleasures. But sometimes, it's good to eat in silence. Focus your thoughts on the flavour, texture and smell of your food. If you find your mind wandering, bring it back to the moment. If you always eat dinner as a family, you could suggest eating in silence for five minutes.

CHECK-IN

Before finishing your plateful or helping yourself to seconds, take a moment to ask yourself if you're still hungry. Has your body had enough to eat? If the answer is yes, don't be afraid to leave what's left on your plate, or save it for later.

SIT DOWN!

Always eating on the go? Set aside some time to sit down and eat your meal or snack, even if it's just 10 minutes. It's hard to appreciate your food and your body's signals when you are multi-tasking. When you sit down, you'll digest your food better too.

TURN OFF THE TV

If TV dinners are the norm for you, chances are you're not registering much of what you eat. The same goes for eating in front of your laptop or at your desk. Put down that phone too!

TAKE A PAUSE

Rather than cramming in the next forkful of food, take a breath to savour the mouthful you've just eaten. You could even try putting down your cutlery at intervals throughout your meal and taking a pause from eating.

Day 13

MAKE TIME FOR FIVE MINUTES OF MEDITATION EACH DAY, STARTING TODAY. SIT IN YOUR QUIET SPOT, IN THE POSITION YOU'VE FOUND TO BE COMFORTABLE, AND SET A TIMER ON YOUR PHONE (PUT IT INTO FLIGHT MODE SO YOU DON'T GET DISTRACTED WITH ALERTS). ALLOW YOUR EYES TO CLOSE OR JUST FOCUS GENTLY ON SOMETHING IN FRONT OF YOU. BEGIN BY PAYING ATTENTION TO YOUR BREATH. DON'T TRY TO CHANGE THE WAY YOU BREATHE — SIMPLY NOTICE IT WITHOUT JUDGEMENT. FEEL YOUR CHEST RISE AND FALL, NOTICE THE COOL AIR GOING IN THROUGH YOUR NOSE AND THE WARMER AIR COMING BACK OUT. NOTICE OTHER SENSATIONS IN YOUR BODY. THOUGHTS WILL BUBBLE UP — THAT'S COMPLETELY NORMAL — BUT RATHER THAN ENGAGING WITH THEM BY TRYING TO PUSH THEM AWAY, SIMPLY ALLOW THEM TO PASS, LIKE CLOUDS ACROSS THE SKY.

HOW I FELT

TODAY'S MINDFUL MOMENTS

Day 14

PLANT SOMETHING. IT CAN BE OUTSIDE IN YOUR GARDEN, IF YOU HAVE ONE, OR INDOORS. TAKE TIME SOWING THE SEEDS, GENTLY COVERING THEM WITH SOIL, THEN WATERING THEM. GARDENING IS A NATURALLY MINDFUL ACTIVITY SO, IF YOU FEEL RELAXED DOING THIS, YOU CAN BUILD ON IT AND GRADUALLY START TO PLANT MORE.

HOW I FELT

TODAY'S MINDFUL MOMENTS

Day 15

NEED TO CLEAR YOUR MIND AT WORK? YOU DON'T NEED TO SET ASIDE 30 MINUTES TO SIT SOMEWHERE QUIET (LET'S FACE IT, WHO CAN MANAGE THAT?) INSTEAD, MAKE A DECISION TO CARRY OUT YOUR NEXT TASK MINDFULLY. TAKE A FEW BREATHS BEFORE YOU BEGIN AND THEN IMMERSE YOURSELF IN THE TASK FOR FIVE MINUTES. FOR EXAMPLE, IF YOU'RE DOING SOME FILING, DON'T GLANCE AT YOUR COMPUTER OR SPEAK TO COLLEAGUES – FOCUS FULLY ON THE FILING. IF YOU'RE WRITING AN EMAIL, CONCENTRATE COMPLETELY ON THAT. YOU'LL PROBABLY FIND YOU DO THE JOB MUCH MORE EFFICIENTLY AND FEEL LESS STRESSED.

HOW I FELT

TODAY'S MINDFUL MOMENTS

MINDFULNESS
FOR KIDS

It's not just you who can benefit from practising mindfulness, your children can reap rewards too. Uz Afazl, mindfulness coach and author of *Mindfulness for Children* (Kyle Books, £14.99) explains how

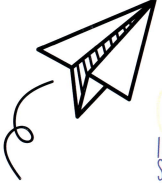

WHAT ARE THE BENEFITS OF MINDFULNESS FOR CHILDREN?

'In today's fast-paced world, it's increasingly tricky for children to focus and simply "be". Mindfulness can help them to deal with the inevitable ups and downs of life. As mindfulness teacher, Jon Kabat-Zinn, says, "You can't stop the waves, but you can learn to surf." Mindfulness gives children a valuable tool they can use to support them when the "waves of life" get choppy.

'It can be a tool to help them calm themselves when they find themselves going into "fight-flight-freeze" reactive mode and give them the space they need to take a more measured approach. It can also help children to slow down and appreciate the experiences they're having.

'A review of the research into mindfulness with children and young people, conducted by Southampton University, found that short, focused sessions of mindfulness in school proved popular with children and teachers and positively impacted on the children's psychological, social and physical wellbeing and flourishing. There also seemed to be a small positive impact on cognition.'

IS MINDFULNESS BEING INTRODUCED TO SCHOOLS?

'There are a number of excellent mindfulness-based initiatives. A few of the most popular ones are the Mindfulness in Schools Programme – Dot B and Paws B. Also, the MindUP programme, developed by Goldie Hawn, which has neuroscience, mindfulness, positive psychology and social and emotional learning at its core. All the children and adults in a school stop three times a day and take a 'brain break' – a short break during which they focus on the sound of a chime and on their breathing. I'm a MindUP consultant and I love going into schools and sharing the programme. It's incredible on follow-up visits to see children as young as three getting involved.'

WHAT ARE THE BENEFITS FOR FAMILY LIFE?

'Children tell me it helps them with their relationships with siblings, with the stresses and anxieties around homework and tests. One parent told me she had so much going on she ended up snapping at her children. Then she noticed one of her sons had taken himself off and was sitting quietly with his eyes closed. He explained that he was practising mindfulness to help him feel calmer. The parent gathered the family together and asked her son to teach them this practice, so they could all benefit from the calm feelings.'

TIPS FOR GETTING STARTED

1 Start with yourself
The in-flight safety advice "Put your own oxygen mask on first before helping anyone else" is as true for mindfulness as for anything else. Start by developing a practice of your own so you have a real and embodied appreciation for it, to pass on to your children.

2 Start small
Try just 30 seconds to a minute (depending on the age and concentration levels of your child) and once they are comfortable with this, gradually increase the time.

3 Have fun
It's not meant to be a chore. Mindfulness can help us when we're experiencing challenges, but it can also help us to live life more deeply and appreciate even the small things.

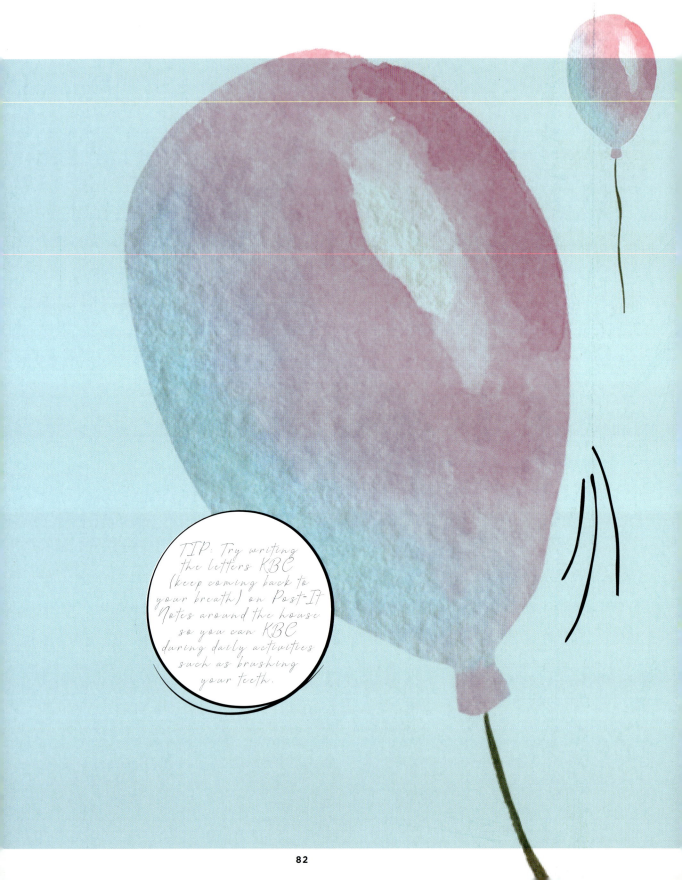

TIP: Try writing the letters KBC (keep coming back to your breath) on Post-It Notes around the house so you can KBC during daily activities such as brushing your teeth.

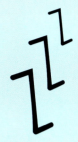

Know children who could benefit from mindfulness? Here are two exercises to try

BALLOON BREATHING

This is a really helpful practice you can use at any time of the day to calm down and focus. It takes one to five minutes, depending on your child's age and ability to concentrate. All you need is your breathing body, a bell or chime (optional).

Read this script to your child. After a number of attempts they may be able to lead themselves in the practice without your support.

● Take a seat. Feel where your feet touch the floor, feel your back straightening and close your eyes or lower your gaze. (If you have a bell or chime, ring it once. Listen to the sound until it fades away. If not, move straight on to the next step.)

● Place your hand on your belly. Imagine you have a small balloon in your belly and each time you breathe in, the balloon blows up, and each time you breathe out, the balloon deflates.

● Feel your belly rising and falling as the balloon blows up and deflates. You don't need to change your breathing or breathe in any special kind of way, just allow your body to breathe freely and naturally.

● As you breathe in, you can say to yourself in your head, 'Blow up balloon' and, as you breathe out, you can say, 'Let all the air out'. Perhaps you can picture the balloon blowing up and deflating with each in- and out-breath. (If you find these words too long, you could shorten them to, 'Blow up' on the in-breath and, 'Air out' on the out-breath.)

Continue for about 30 seconds to three minutes, depending on the child's age and attention span. Repeat the guiding words to support your child's focus, leaving some brief periods of silence (five to 10 seconds) in between. About halfway through the practice, say this next line.

● If your mind wanders off into thoughts, that's okay, gently bring your focus back to your breath. (At the end of the practice, if you have a bell or chime, ring it once. Listen to the sound of the bell. Wait for 10 seconds.)

● Gently open your eyes or raise your gaze.

After the practice, you can ask your child what they noticed or felt as they practised. Whatever they report, acknowledge that it was good that they noticed their experience, as that's mindfulness. Remind them it's okay if their mind wandered and give them encouragement if they remembered to KBC (keep coming back) to their breath.

TAKE FIVE

This practice can help your child to notice what they have to be grateful for in a day. It's nice if you finish by sharing with your child one thing about them that makes you feel grateful. It takes one minute and all you need is you.

Read this introduction to your child the first few times you practise.

● Being thankful can help you to feel happier, so this is a nice practice to end the day.

Read this practice script to your child. After a number of attempts they may be able to lead themselves in the practice without your support.

● Think about, or say aloud, one thing you are thankful for from today, such as having a good friend, eating a delicious meal, playing in the sun or the rain, reading a good book, having a loving family, and count this on one finger.

● Think of another thing you are thankful for from today, and count this on another finger.

● Keep going until you've counted out thanks on all five fingers.

● And now, here's one thing about you that made me feel thankful today... Good night.

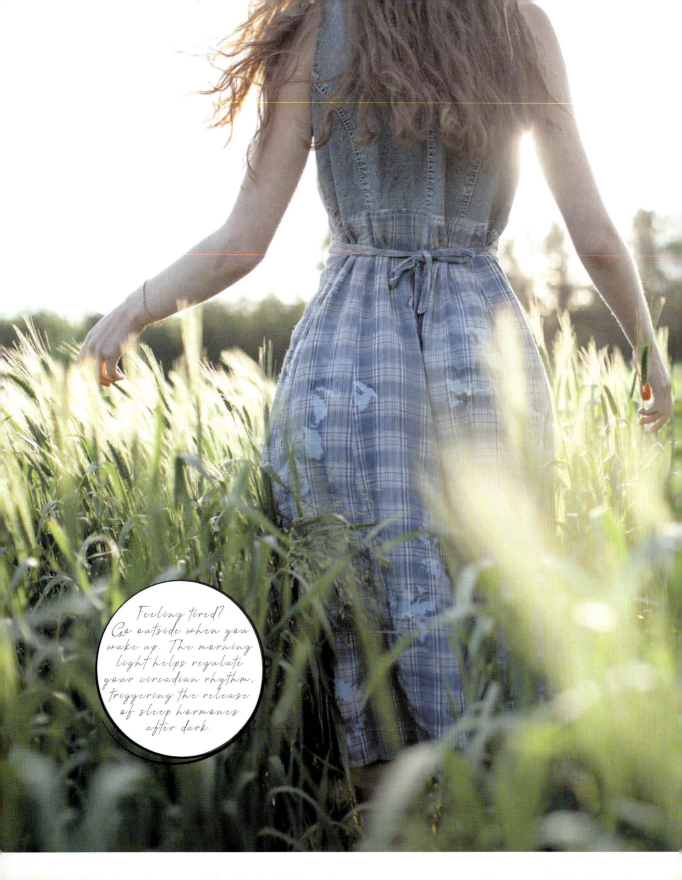

Feeling tired?
Go outside when you
wake up. The morning
light helps regulate
your circadian rhythm,
triggering the release
of sleep hormones
after dark.

PRESS PAUSE

Does your life feel it's spinning out of control? Here's how to recapture your natural rhythm

Do you stay up too late watching TV? Do you get woken every morning by the buzz of your alarm? Modern day 24/7 living means we can lose our connection to more natural rhythms. Tuning into your body on a regular basis to discover what it needs will bring you back into a more harmonious rhythm, freeing up your energy and leaving you feeling happy and optimistic.

TRY THIS

1 Find a place in nature that you love, ideally with water nearby, and ban all technology.

2 Spend the next hour considering a 'big' question in your life – what you long for, need or who you truly are.

3 Breathe deeply and let your imagination wander, allowing insights to come to you rather than using your logic.

'The body benefits from movement, and the mind benefits from stillness'

SAKYANG MIPHAM

MOVING
MEDITATION

Still struggling to clear your mind or can't sit still long enough to meditate? Getting active could be your short-cut to calm. In this section, we explain how exercise and activity can bring you into the moment. Discover how to get 'in the zone' like an athlete and boost your performance. Take a mindful walk or run, and try a meditative yin yoga sequence that will boost your body while it soothes your mind.

Day 16

TURN TIDYING INTO A MINDFUL ACTIVITY. CHOOSE ONE SHELF OR DRAWER IN YOUR HOME AND CLEAR EVERYTHING FROM IT. CLEAN THE SHELF OR DRAWER CAREFULLY. THEN DECIDE WHAT YOU WANT TO PUT BACK IN BY PICKING UP EACH OBJECT YOU REMOVED, LOOKING AT IT AND FEELING IT. NOTICE EVERYTHING ABOUT IT BEFORE YOU PUT IT BACK OR DECIDE TO LEAVE IT OUT.

HOW I FELT

TODAY'S MINDFUL MOMENTS

Day 17

HAVE A SOUND MIND! CHOOSE A TUNE YOU LOVE AND SIT QUIETLY WHILE LISTENING TO IT. IT MAY BE HELPFUL TO CLOSE YOUR EYES. USUALLY, WE HAVE MUSIC ON IN THE BACKGROUND SO WE DON'T GIVE IT OUR FULL ATTENTION. NOTICE EVERYTHING ABOUT THE TUNE, FROM ANY LYRICS TO THE BEAT AND THE INSTRUMENTS YOU CAN HEAR BEING PLAYED. ONCE THE MUSIC IS FINISHED, JOT DOWN ANYTHING YOU PICKED UP THAT YOU DON'T NORMALLY HEAR WHEN YOU LISTEN TO THIS PIECE OF MUSIC.

HOW I FELT

TODAY'S MINDFUL MOMENTS

Day 18

TAKE A SHOWER WITH PRESENCE. IT'S A BIT OF QUIET TIME MOST OF US HAVE EVERY MORNING SO MAXIMISE THE BENEFITS BY MAKING IT MINDFUL. TAKE A MOMENT TO ASSEMBLE EVERYTHING YOU'LL NEED FOR YOUR SHOWER. WHEN YOU'RE READY, GET IN. PAY ATTENTION TO THE SENSATION OF THE WATER RUNNING OVER YOUR SKIN. INHALE THE STEAM AND THE SCENT OF THE SOAP YOU'RE USING, PICKING UP ON ALL THE DIFFERENT NOTES. FULLY EXPERIENCE THE FEELING OF THE SOAP ON YOUR SKIN, AND ANY BRUSH OR BODY SCRUB YOU'RE USING. WHEN YOU'RE READY, TURN THE SHOWER OFF AND NOTICE THE COOLER AIR ON YOUR BODY AS YOU GET OUT. DRY YOURSELF MINDFULLY, CAREFULLY TOWELLING EVERY PART OF YOU.

HOW I FELT

TODAY'S MINDFUL MOMENTS

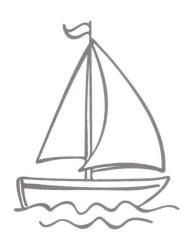

MOVE YOUR MIND

Find it hard to switch off? Turn your workouts into a mindfulness session and boost your performance while you relax your mind

If you find it hard to sit still - not to mention clear your mind – moving your body can help transport you into a mindful state. Whether it's the beat of your feet hitting the pavement as you walk or the sound of your breathing as you run, rhythmic forms of exercise can induce you into a state of 'flow' where, absorbed in the activity, your body and mind work in harmony and all other thoughts fall away. Athletes call it 'being in the zone' but you can also call it mindfulness.

Indeed, studies conducted on runners and athletes when they're 'in the zone', show their brain waves are similar to those that occur during a meditative state. It's a state of mind and body where performance becomes effortless, races are won and medals broken. It's also one of the reasons why so many successful entrepreneurs, artists and writers make

exercise a non-negotiable part of their daily life. It refreshes your brain and helps ideas flow and productivity sky rocket.

THINK TO WIN

Do you rely on running as a way to resolve your problems, or have a swim after work to relax your mind at the end of a busy week? You're already experiencing the benefits of moving meditation. But, by applying some mindfulness techniques to your workout sessions, you can multiply the mental benefits.

On a physical level, sports science shows that staying mindful while you workout not only reduces injury but improves the body benefits and boosts performance. Many sports coaches now employ mindfulness as part of their athletes' training programmes.

THE MINDFUL WORKOUT

Here's how to make your next workout session more mindful.

1. During your warm-up, tune into your body. How does it feel – is it slow and tired or raring to go?

2. Pay attention to any muscle that feels tight or joint that feels stiff. Close your eyes and breathe into the area, letting go of any pain or discomfort as you exhale.

3. Once you start to workout, avoid the

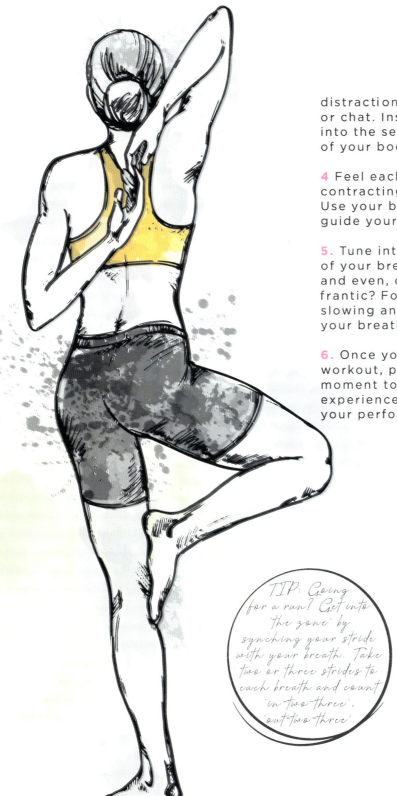

distractions of TV, music or chat. Instead, tune into the sensations of your body.

4 Feel each muscle contracting as it works. Use your breath to guide your efforts.

5. Tune into the rhythm of your breath. Is it deep and even, or shallow and frantic? Focus on slowing and deepening your breath.

6. Once you finish your workout, pause for a moment to absorb the experience and review your performance.

TIP: Going for a run? Get into 'the zone' by synching your stride with your breath. Take two or three strides to each breath and count 'in-two-three', 'out-two-three'.

'IT WORKS FOR ME'
Jessica Robson
Founder of RunTalkRun

'Running really helps my anxiety. It brings me back to my breath and to a calmer state. I tried meditation but found I'm better at it when I'm on the move. Sometimes I go out and it's about being aware of my breath, other days I time it with the rhythm of my feet. At the start of a run, I'm quite pent up but by the end, I feel much calmer and more free. I think it's the mindfulness of being outside and being aware of something bigger than what's in my head.

'I was having therapy for struggles with my mental health but found I was opening up more freely when running with my mum – it was less intimidating. So I started RunTalkRun sessions to offer a relaxed, safe space where people can run and open up.'
Visit runtalkrun.com; @runtalkrun

WALK INTO
WISDOM

Walking meditation is a classic mindfulness exercise that can enhance your daily life

indful walking is a simple way of going on a journey with yourself, using the rhythm of your footsteps and your breath to bring you into awareness. Usually, when we walk, we're rushing from A to B, chatting with friends or mulling over problems. But walking in the present moment, paying attention to the sensations of your body and surroundings, helps develop your sense of self and your connection to the environment.

TIP: Use mindful walking as a stand-alone practice or add it into your daily life whenever you're feeling stressed.

1. Find a clear, quiet space to walk. If you're indoors you can walk in circles.

2. Stand still, your arms relaxed by your sides. Feel your feet in contact with the ground, your legs rooted, your body tall. Sway your body slightly until you find your ideal balance.

3. Tune into your breath and focus on your breathing for a minute or two.

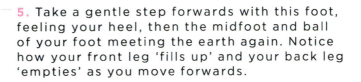

4. Take your attention to your feet. Gently shift your weight onto one foot and gently raise the heel of your opposite foot, peeling it away from the ground. Take in the sensation, moving slowly and purposefully.

5. Take a gentle step forwards with this foot, feeling your heel, then the midfoot and ball of your foot meeting the earth again. Notice how your front leg 'fills up' and your back leg 'empties' as you move forwards.

6. Now take a second step with your opposite leg and continue to walk forwards, staying tuned to the sensations in your feet, legs and body, the swaying of your hips, the tensing and releasing of the muscles in your legs.

7. When you come to the end of your walk, bring your back foot to meet your front foot and pause, witnessing the stillness. Then turn around, re-centre yourself and walk back in the other direction.

TIP: Walking barefoot helps heighten the experience of your meditation.

TUNE IN

As you walk, it's likely that thoughts will come and go. Simply turn your attention back to walking and to your breath. To stay focused, try counting your steps or saying 'stepping' for each step or 'left', 'right'. Or use the rhythm of your breath to regulate your steps. Once you're accustomed to the practice, you can work mindful walking into your life, adapting your practice to bring variety and help you connect to your surroundings. You could try switching your attention between your body and the sensations around you – the scent of flowers and freshly cut grass, the crunch of leaves, or the feel of rain on your face.

ON THE

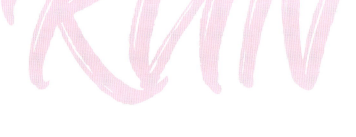

Beat stress, boost recovery and feel happy by making your running more mindful

If you're a runner, you might already be familiar with one of the great pluses of combining running with mindfulness – being in the "flow state", says William Pullen, psychotherapist and author of *Run For Your Life* (Penguin Books, £9.99) . 'This powerful sensation is a kind of mental state that comes from feeling completely immersed in and absorbed by an activity you enjoy. Mindful running is the practice of immersing yourself in your physical experience of the world around, substituting thoughts of the past and future with the sensations of the here and now.

'Mindful running is particularly effective because the process of running itself keeps your mind involved in a way that sitting often doesn't. You're not left with that extra brain power that can leave you self-conscious or ruminating when you're at rest. Instead, when you run, your body/mind is kept occupied at just the right level, leaving you free to fully focus on the changing environment around you.'

1. Find a green space you are reasonably familiar with.

2. Take a couple of deep breaths and remind yourself why you are there.

3. Focus on the sensation of the world carrying your weight, try to really plant yourself where you are.

4. Begin running slowly. Remember this is not about distance or speed.

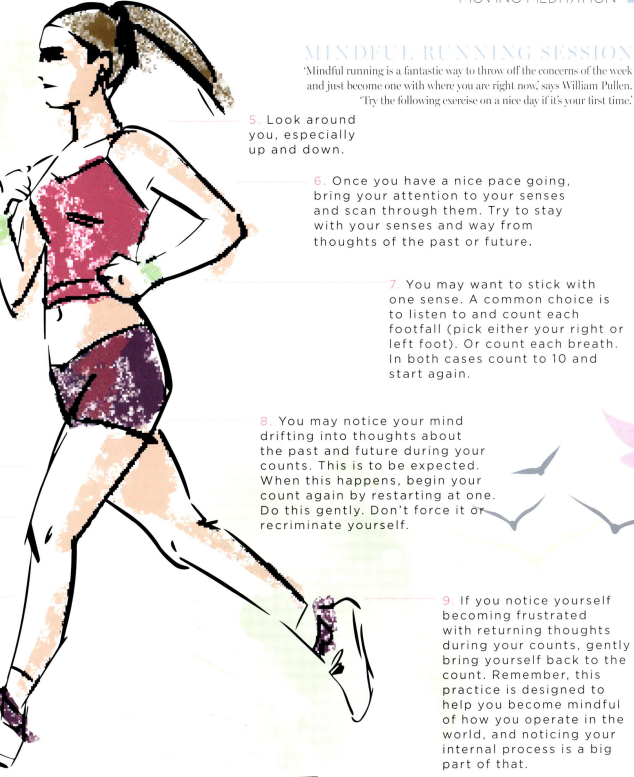

MINDFUL RUNNING SESSION

'Mindful running is a fantastic way to throw off the concerns of the week and just become one with where you are right now,' says William Pullen. 'Try the following exercise on a nice day if it's your first time.'

5. Look around you, especially up and down.

6. Once you have a nice pace going, bring your attention to your senses and scan through them. Try to stay with your senses and way from thoughts of the past or future.

7. You may want to stick with one sense. A common choice is to listen to and count each footfall (pick either your right or left foot). Or count each breath. In both cases count to 10 and start again.

8. You may notice your mind drifting into thoughts about the past and future during your counts. This is to be expected. When this happens, begin your count again by restarting at one. Do this gently. Don't force it or recriminate yourself.

9. If you notice yourself becoming frustrated with returning thoughts during your counts, gently bring yourself back to the count. Remember, this practice is designed to help you become mindful of how you operate in the world, and noticing your internal process is a big part of that.

FLEX YOUR MIND

Fusing body and mind, yoga poses are naturally mindful. Here's how to deepen your experience

By its very definition, yoga is mindfulness in action. Its name in Sanskrit means 'to yoke' or 'union', a reference to the fusing of body and mind. This ancient system of exercise uses the breath to guide the body through a series of asanas (poses) that work on all the body's systems and organs, to bring it into balance. As you absorb yourself in each asana, you automatically come into the present moment, forgetting everyday thoughts and focusing only on the here and now of your body and breath. Many systems of yoga incorporate meditation and breathwork to further deepen the experience.

BE MINDFUL

These days, yoga classes often focus more on the physical, athletic side of yoga, providing more of a workout for your body than your mind. But if you're feeling stressed or want to balance your other workouts, it's worth trying a few different classes to find a more mindful experience or create your own practice.

'Doing asanas without mindfulness is gymnastics. That's all good – it still benefits your body – but if we leave out the mind, we rob ourselves of something very precious – the conscious connection to presence, the source of life', says Esther Ekhart founder of EkhartYoga. 'Yoga points to stillness and bringing the frustrations of the mind to stillness so, if that's your goal and you want to do yoga the way it was meant to be, you have to bring in mindfulness.'

Here are some tips to make your yoga classes an even more mindful experience. Take a few moments to absorb the experience and any insights that arise.

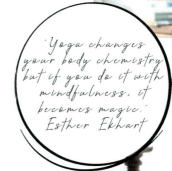

'Yoga changes your body chemistry but if you do it with mindfulness, it becomes magic.'
Esther Ekhart

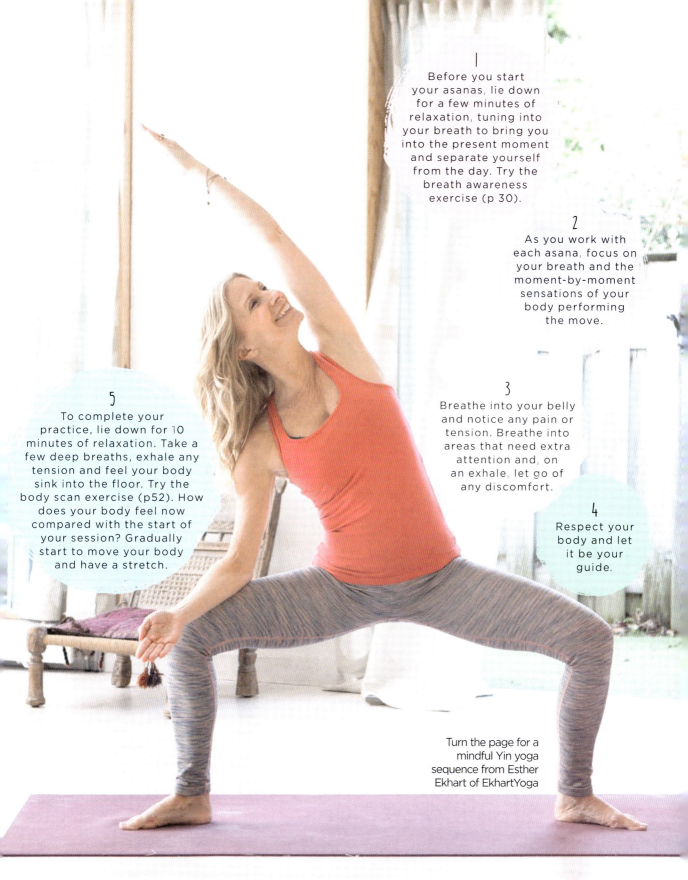

1
Before you start your asanas, lie down for a few minutes of relaxation, tuning into your breath to bring you into the present moment and separate yourself from the day. Try the breath awareness exercise (p 30).

2
As you work with each asana, focus on your breath and the moment-by-moment sensations of your body performing the move.

3
Breathe into your belly and notice any pain or tension. Breathe into areas that need extra attention and, on an exhale, let go of any discomfort.

4
Respect your body and let it be your guide.

5
To complete your practice, lie down for 10 minutes of relaxation. Take a few deep breaths, exhale any tension and feel your body sink into the floor. Try the body scan exercise (p52). How does your body feel now compared with the start of your session? Gradually start to move your body and have a stretch.

Turn the page for a mindful Yin yoga sequence from Esther Ekhart of EkhartYoga

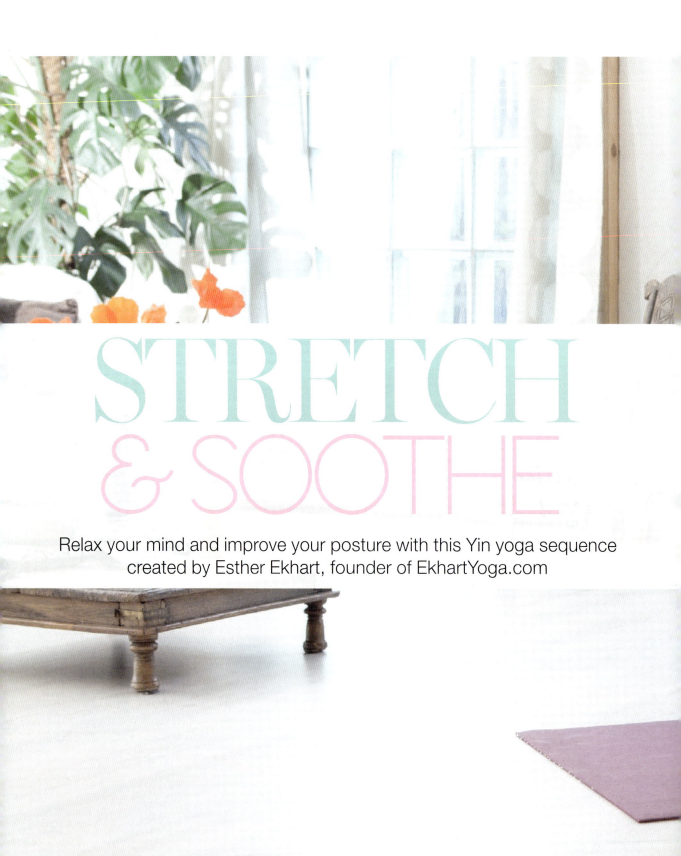

STRETCH
& SOOTHE

Relax your mind and improve your posture with this Yin yoga sequence
created by Esther Ekhart, founder of EkhartYoga.com

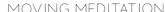

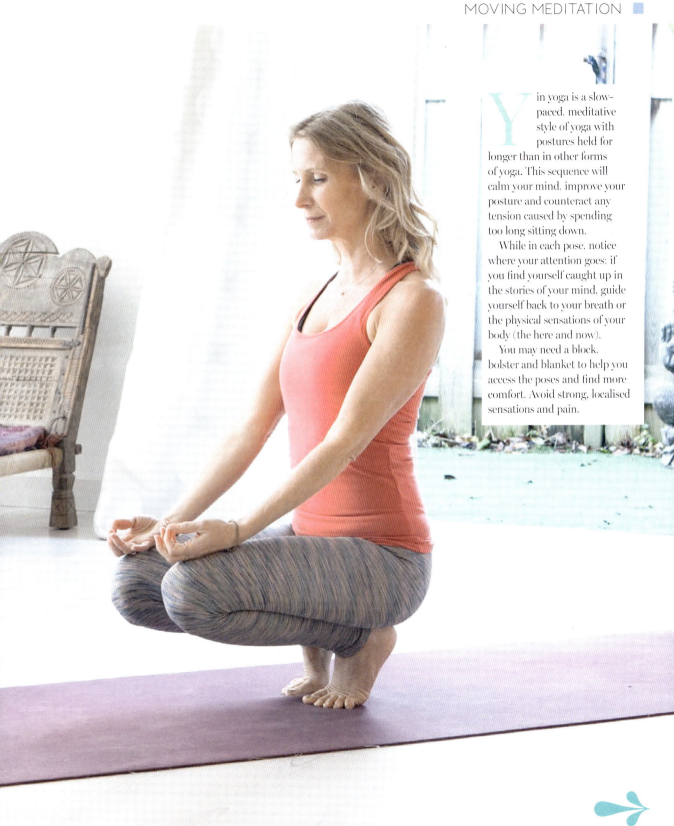

Yin yoga is a slow-paced, meditative style of yoga with postures held for longer than in other forms of yoga. This sequence will calm your mind, improve your posture and counteract any tension caused by spending too long sitting down.

While in each pose, notice where your attention goes: if you find yourself caught up in the stories of your mind, guide yourself back to your breath or the physical sensations of your body (the here and now).

You may need a block, bolster and blanket to help you access the poses and find more comfort. Avoid strong, localised sensations and pain.

TOE SQUAT

This is a great pose to stretch your toes and stimulate your lower-body meridians. It can be quite challenging, though, so rest your hands on the floor, or blocks, if needed.

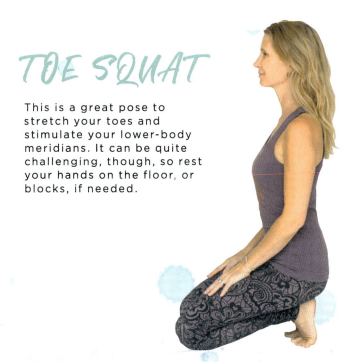

First, sit on your heels with your feet together, then bring your weight forwards and tuck all your toes under, including your little toes. Now, try to bring most of your weight back to the balls of your feet. Breathe and observe your mind's reaction to the sensations, which can be pretty intense!

You can stay in this pose for 30 seconds and up to three minutes.

SPHINX POSE

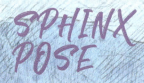

This pose will help you to restore the natural curvature in your lumbar spine and promote tissue regeneration in your sacrum area. Like many backbends, this pose will also leave you feeling energised.

Lie on your stomach, legs a comfortable distance apart, and bring your elbows more or less under your shoulders. Place a bolster under your ribs for support and allow your buttocks to relax.

Stay in this pose for three to five minutes.

MELTING HEART

This is a wonderful posture for counteracting a slumped, rounded spine, and creating space in your chest and sides of your body.

From your hands and knees, lower down onto your elbows, bringing your palms to touch and keeping your hips in line with your knees. Rest your forehead on a block or the floor and, as you breathe, try to relax and soften your chest area. Use a bolster to support your chest if needed.

Stay in the pose for one to three minutes.

SUPPORTED BRIDGE

Another gentle backbend, this pose will help you revitalise your adrenal glands and ground your energy.

Lie on your back, bend your knees and place your feet parallel to each other, a comfortable distance away from your hips. Inhale and gently press your feet down to lift your hips up and bring your shoulder blades towards each other. Place a block under your sacrum and lower your hips down.

Allow your breath to move towards your belly while staying in this pose for three to five minutes.

RECLINED TWIST

This gentle twist is great for restoring spine neutrality and bringing your nervous system back into balance.

Lie on your back, move your hips a little over to the right and bring your knees over to the left. Support your knees with a block or a bolster. Gaze upwards or turn your head to the right.
   You can stay in this twist for three to five minutes, breathing fully and evenly, then repeat on the other side.

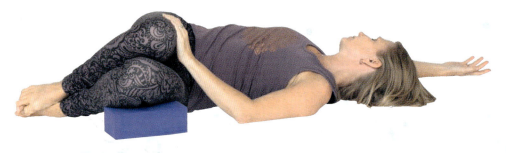

DRAGONFLY

This posture stretches your inner thighs and stimulates your spleen meridian. As it can be a challenging pose, use it is an opportunity to work with the spleen energy, which is about acceptance.

Sit on a cushion or a folded blanket, ground your sitting bones and take your legs out wide. Keeping your spine long, begin to fold forwards from your hips. Depending on your range of movement, use your arms, blocks or a bolster to support your upper body. Hold this pose for three to five minutes.

HAPPY BABY

This pose is wonderful for increasing hip mobility and helps to decompress the sacroiliac joint.

DRAGONFLY WITH SIDE BEND

This pose will give you a lateral flexion of your spine and stimulate your gall bladder meridian, which is linked to discernment and healthy choices.

From a seated position, take your legs wide apart, and then ground your sitting bones to find length in your spine. If you find your pelvis tilting backwards, sit up on a couple of folded blankets. Bend sideways and rest your elbow on a block so you can support your head in your hand. If comfortable to do so, you can gently rotate your chest towards the ceiling.

You can stay here for up to three minutes, then repeat on the other side.

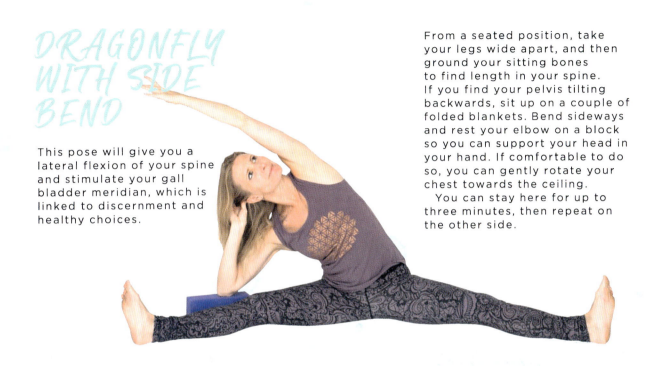

RECLINED BUTTERFLY

Lying on your back, hug your knees to your chest and hold the outer edges of your feet or ankles with your hands. Bring your feet over your knees and gently press your knees towards the floor. You can stay still or gently rock from side to side, massaging your lower back. Stay in this pose for up to three minutes.

This posture rejuvenates the body and calms the mind. It's a lovely pose to incorporate at the end of your practice to observe the space you've created, physically and mentally.

Lie down on your back, with a bolster underneath your knees. Bring the soles of your feet together and allow your knees to fall out to the sides. Let your body relax fully and deeply, and breathe… Enjoy it for five to 15 minutes.

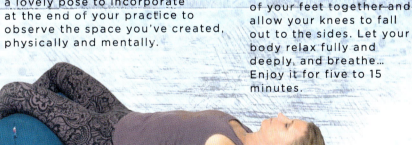

For online yoga and meditation classes, visit ekhartyoga.com/classes

Day 19

GO WITH THE FLOW WHILE YOU'RE ON THE MOVE. SEE THOSE TRANSPORT DELAYS AND TRAFFIC JAMS AS GOOD OPPORTUNITIES TO PRACTISE A SPOT OF MINDFULNESS. WHEN YOU'RE STUCK ON A TRAIN OR WAITING AT A RED LIGHT, FOCUS ON YOUR POSTURE. ARE YOU SITTING AS COMFORTABLY AS POSSIBLE? BRING YOUR ATTENTION TO YOUR BREATHING. EVEN IF IT'S ONLY FOR A MOMENT OR TWO, IT ALL COUNTS.

HOW I FELT

TODAY'S MINDFUL MOMENTS

Day 20

FIX SOMETHING. FIND SOMETHING THAT NEEDS MENDING – WHETHER IT'S A HEM THAT NEEDS TO BE STITCHED OR A VASE THAT'S CRACKED – AND ASSEMBLE EVERYTHING YOU NEED TO MEND IT. TAKE YOUR TIME, CAREFULLY MAKING THE REPAIR. DO IT AS SLOWLY AS YOU CAN, FOCUSING CLOSELY ON WHAT YOU'RE DOING. PAY ATTENTION TO THE PROCESS. NOTICE THE FEEL OF THE ITEM IN YOUR HANDS, THE SENSATIONS IN YOUR BODY AS YOU CONCENTRATE AND THE FEELING OF SATISFACTION YOU GET WHEN THE JOB IS COMPLETE.

HOW I FELT

TODAY'S MINDFUL MOMENTS

Day 21

WANT TO SLEEP WELL TONIGHT? USE THIS YIN YOGA POSE TO GET INTO A MINDFUL PLACE. TRY LYING DOWN WITH YOUR LEGS RESTING AGAINST A WALL FOR FIVE MINUTES. WHILE YOU'RE LYING THERE, BRING YOUR FOCUS TO YOUR BREATH AND TO THE PHYSICAL SENSE OF DEEP RELAXATION. THIS IS A GREAT ONE TO PRACTISE JUST BEFORE BED.

HOW I FELT

TODAY'S MINDFUL MOMENTS

'Much of spiritual life is self-acceptance, maybe all of it'

JACK KORNFIELD

MINDFUL THERAPY

When was the last occasion you had a good belly laugh or allowed yourself time to play? Mindfulness isn't just about slowing down and meditating. In this chapter, we celebrate the many ways you can naturally connect with the moment and discover your inner joy. Discover why gratitude can make you happier; tap into your spirituality to boost your health; and make a vision board to help turn your dreams into reality.

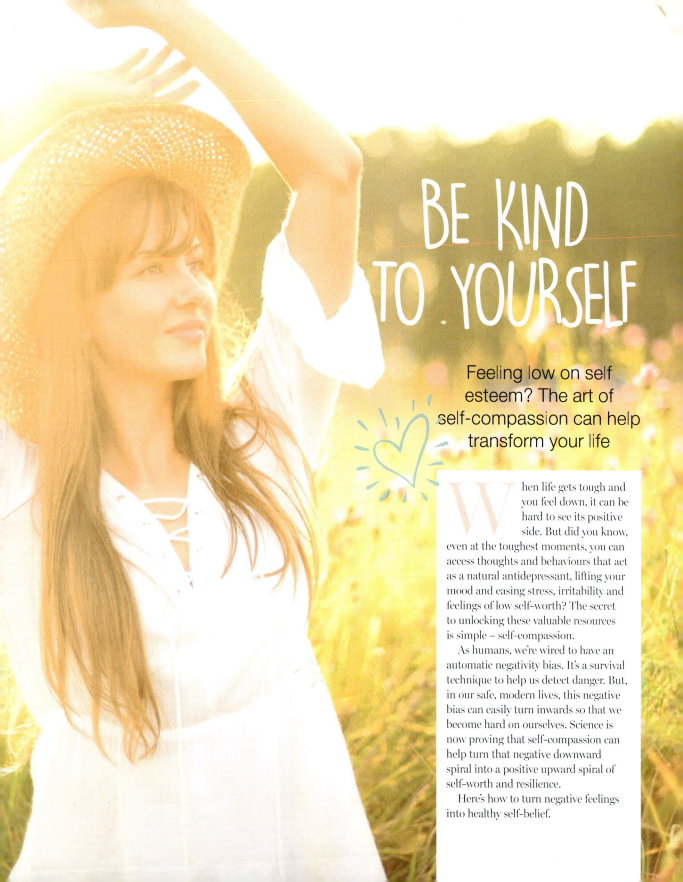

BE KIND TO YOURSELF

Feeling low on self esteem? The art of self-compassion can help transform your life

When life gets tough and you feel down, it can be hard to see its positive side. But did you know, even at the toughest moments, you can access thoughts and behaviours that act as a natural antidepressant, lifting your mood and easing stress, irritability and feelings of low self-worth? The secret to unlocking these valuable resources is simple – self-compassion.

As humans, we're wired to have an automatic negativity bias. It's a survival technique to help us detect danger. But, in our safe, modern lives, this negative bias can easily turn inwards so that we become hard on ourselves. Science is now proving that self-compassion can help turn that negative downward spiral into a positive upward spiral of self-worth and resilience.

Here's how to turn negative feelings into healthy self-belief.

ARE YOU TOO HARD ON YOURSELF?

Tick any of the following that apply:

1. I GET ANGRY WITH MYSELF IF I LOSE MY TEMPER OR FEEL DOWN.

2. WHEN SOMETHING GOES WRONG, I IMMEDIATELY WORRY IT MAY BE MY FAULT.

3. I RUN MYSELF INTO THE GROUND GETTING THINGS DONE FOR OTHER PEOPLE FOR FEAR OF LETTING ANYONE DOWN.

4. TAKING TIME FOR MYSELF FEELS SELF-INDULGENT.

1. RELAX

Nobody's perfect! It's easy to forget this when you're feeling low but everyone is flawed. Remember this fact and you'll start to take your own perceived failings less personally and take care of yourself in challenging moments. 'The vulnerability of our imperfection is the gateway to self-acceptance, self-love, and healing,' says Elisha Goldstein, psychologist and author of *Uncovering Happiness* (Simon & Schuster, £12.99).

2. MAKE TIME FOR YOURSELF

In difficult moments, take some time out for a self-compassion break. Place your hand on your heart and say, 'May I be at ease' (or happy, healthy, free from fear – whatever you need at that moment). You can also use this time to send good wishes to people in your life.

3. TAKE COMFORT

Need a hug? Showing yourself a little kindness triggers the release of oxytocin – the 'love hormone'. It's also triggered by cuddling, breast feeding and falling in love. 'This biochemical response is the opposite of what happens when we're caught in the depression loop,' says Goldstein. 'Engaging in self-compassion changes your brain chemistry.'

4. HUG IT OUT

If you have someone around, give them a long meaningful hug. Let it linger – it's doing you good! 'If you don't have someone at home, imagine hugging another person, hug yourself, or set the intention to hug others more often,' says Goldstein. 'In doing this, you're nurturing the release of this natural antidepressant.'

5. FIND YOUR BALANCE

The higher our stress levels are, the more fear we have. Self-compassion dissolves both. And you're not just doing it for yourself. Self-compassion and self-love will improve your relationships with those around you. So remember self-compassion is not self-indulgence!

BE SAFE

DREAM ON

Don't feel guilty if you let your mind wander sometimes… it has a wealth of wellbeing benefits

Daydreaming gets a bad rap. We tend to associate it with being vague and fanciful. Perhaps you were told off for daydreaming at school and, as an adult, you make an effort not to let your mind drift so you seem more purposeful and serious. Yet research shows that when your mind wanders, your brain recruits complex areas including the region associated with problem solving. And in two studies from the University of Central Lancashire, researchers found that far from being a distraction, daydreaming can help you become more creative. When you're in a state of 'passive boredom', for instance when your mind drifts off in a dull meeting, your mind switches to creative lateral thinking and comes up with ideas.

Here's how to get the benefits:

TRY SELF HYPNOSIS

If you're in a job that overstimulates you, try this exercise. Lie down, close your eyes and relax your muscles, then allow your mind to wander for 10 minutes.

LET YOUR MIND DRIFT

On a train or bus journey, resist reading your phone or a book. Let your mind wander instead.

TAKE ON BORING JOBS

Rather than putting off the filing or mowing the lawn, embrace those tasks. Make time every day to do a job that bores you, and don't rush it!

TURN THE TV OFF

At home, do the ironing or washing up without the radio or TV on. Yes it makes the job more boring – but that's the point! You'll be surprised how quickly the task passes – in a daydream state your sense of time is less acute.

It's important to bore yourself from time to time in order to stir the creative part of your brain.

Day 22

DO SOME BAKING. IT'S ANOTHER GREAT MINDFUL ACTIVITY. CHOOSE A RECIPE AND GET ALL THE INGREDIENTS READY. GIVE YOURSELF PLENTY OF TIME AND MAKE SURE YOU WON'T BE DISTURBED, SO YOU DON'T HAVE TO RUSH ANYTHING. ENSURE YOUR KITCHEN'S CLEAN AND QUIET AND TURN OFF THE RADIO. NOW, GO THROUGH THE RECIPE ONE STEP AT A TIME, METHODICALLY. FOLLOW EACH STEP SLOWLY AND CAREFULLY, FROM PREHEATING THE OVEN TO GREASING THE DISH AND MEASURING OUT THE INGREDIENTS. REALLY PAY ATTENTION TO WHAT YOU'RE DOING. BY THE TIME IT'S IN THE OVEN, YOU SHOULD FEEL RELAXED AND REFRESHED, BECAUSE YOU'VE GIVEN YOUR BUSY THOUGHTS A BREAK.

HOW I FELT

TODAY'S MINDFUL MOMENTS

Day 23

KEEP CHECKING IN WITH YOURSELF. THROUGHOUT THE DAY, TAKE A MOMENT EVERY HOUR TO NOTICE HOW YOU ARE. IS YOUR BODY TENSE? IS YOUR BREATHING SHALLOW? IS YOUR MIND WANDERING ONTO MULTIPLE DIFFERENT TASKS AND AWAY FROM THE MOMENT? ASK YOURSELF THESE QUESTIONS AND TAKE A MINUTE TO BRING YOURSELF BACK INTO THE PRESENT AND RELAX. YOU COULD SET AN HOURLY ALARM ON YOUR PHONE.

HOW I FELT

TODAY'S MINDFUL MOMENTS

Day 24

SLOW DOWN AT WORK. EVER HEARD THE EXPRESSION 'MORE HASTE, LESS SPEED'? THIS EXERCISE IS ABOUT TAKING TIME TO DO EVERYTHING THOROUGHLY. WHATEVER YOU'RE DOING, SLOW RIGHT DOWN. BE METICULOUS. THIS CAN FEEL DIFFICULT WHEN YOU'RE BUSY BUT TRY DOING IT FOR HALF AN HOUR AND YOU'LL NOTICE HOW MUCH YOU'VE ACHIEVED.

HOW I FELT

TODAY'S MINDFUL MOMENTS

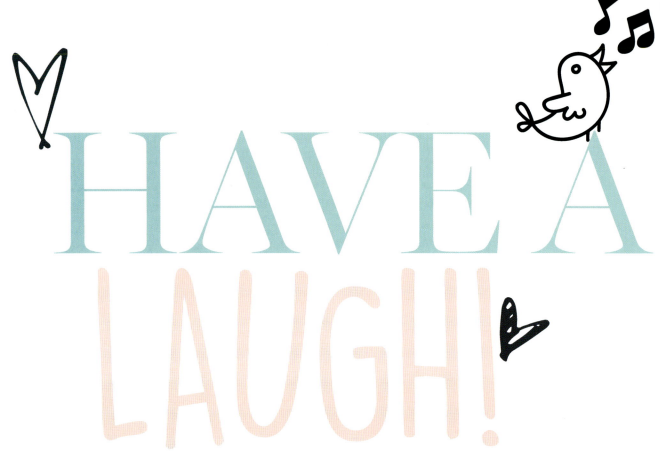

HAVE A LAUGH!

It's time to rediscover one of purest forms of mindfulness – laughter

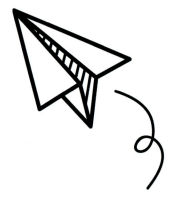

Can you remember the last time you laughed till you cried? You know – one of those belly laughs that makes the tears stream down your face, leaving you struggling to speak. It's a great feeling. That's because laughing releases the feelgood hormone serotonin and alters your brainwaves, clearing your mind and bringing a sense of wellbeing. Laughter boosts your circulation by over 20 per cent, flushing your system with revitalising nutrients and oxygen. And muscle contractions act like a mini workout, releasing tension and boosting lymph flow to strengthen your immune system.

And it's not just your body that benefits. Laughter is a natural form of mindfulness – when you're doubled up in hysterics, everything else is forgotten and you're truly in the moment.

LAUGHTER YOGA

It's said that children laugh more than 300 times a day, but the average 40-year-old laughs just four times a day. But here's the good news – laughter is a skill you can re-learn. And you don't need to hear or watch something funny to do it; you don't even need to be happy. Research shows that doing laughter exercises can give you the same mind and body benefits as spontaneous guffaws. A new breed of yoga therapists and laughter yoga classes use a combination of breath work, playfulness and laughter exercises to help people rediscover their happy place.

Ready to give it a go? Try these tips from laughter therapist Lisa Sturge, author of *Laugh: Everyday Laughter Healing for Greater Happiness and Wellbeing* (Quadrille, £7.99).

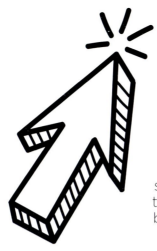

SMILE INSIDE

Stand with your feet hip-width apart, arms at your sides. Breathing slowly, take your attention to the area just below your belly button and imagine a smile there. Connect with this smile and imagine it travelling down your legs to your toes. Picture a smile on the soles of your feet. On an inhale, smile outwardly as you rise onto your toes and bring your arms up as high as is comfortable, then lower your hands and feet as you exhale with an audible sigh: 'haaa'. Repeat a couple of times then stand still, imagining a smile somewhere in your body.

TUMMY LAUGHS

With a partner or a group of friends, lie on your back, with your head on another person's belly and laugh gently.

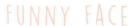

FUNNY FACE

Inhale in front of a mirror or a friend and, as you exhale, make funny faces using sound if you wish. You can also use your hands to help contort your face.

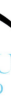

DID YOU KNOW?

A good laugh triggers gamma brainwaves similar to those released by meditation.

PLAY TIME

Want to be happier and more creative?
Give yourself some time to fool around

Next time you find yourself reading a book when you should be cleaning the house or playing with your cat when you should be going for a run, don't be hard on yourself. Research shows the more childlike we are in our thinking, the more creative we become. Far from mere pleasure, play is key to brain development, making us sharper, more adaptable and empathetic, say scientists. In fact, it has led to some of the world's greatest ideas and inventions.

GAME ON

Want to reap the benefits? According to psychologist Stuart Brown, we all have a particular play personality and type of play that suits us best. Read the descriptions (right) to discover your ideal one. Then, all that's left for you to do is get started, which isn't easy because most of us have play conditioned out of us at a young age. As we get older, we're made to feel guilty for playing and told it's a waste of time when, in fact, free play allows you to be creative and develop new ways of looking at things.

So, give yourself permission to dawdle, daydream, laugh and spend time fooling around – even if you're not achieving anything. Because with every moment, you're improving your brain power, creativity and wellbeing.

WHAT'S YOUR PLAY TYPE?

Read the descriptions and decide which sounds like you. You may relate to elements of several but choose the one that sums you up best. If two types describe you equally well, read the suggestions for both.

THE EXPLORER

You love making new discoveries, whether a new holiday destination, the hottest exercise craze or a new relationship.

Your perfect play: Save up for adventure trips or sign up for a fun new evening class.

THE JOKER

Making people laugh gives you a kick, and you love practical jokes.

Your perfect play: Watching comedies or trying your hand at stand up or entertaining friends.

THE ARTIST

You love making things. Cooking, painting or knitting are your ideal ways to relax.

Your perfect play: Try a new craft.

THE STORYTELLER

You adore reading books and watching films and get caught up in them.

Your perfect play: Try writing short stories, poetry or a novel. Join a writing class or enter a competition.

THE COMPETITOR

You feel great when you win or succeed at something. And you like keeping score.

Your perfect play: Play a team sport, or take up competitive running or cycling. Try mental games such as cards.

THE KINESTHETE

Movement is key to play for you. You feel relaxed when dancing, walking or swimming and you're bursting with energy.

Your perfect play: Playing sport for the fun aspect, rather than the competition.

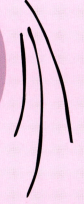

GET CRAFTY

When was the last time you tried making something? It's time to create some happiness

Ever want to break free from your 9-5 and the monotonous routine of the working week? Just as our bodies need exercise breaks, sometimes our brains need a different way to express themselves too. And crafting – creating something unique with your own hands – is the perfect way to do it. As our lives become increasingly tied to technology, it's no surprise that crafts, from knitting and sewing to painting and sculpting, are becoming hugely popular.

THE POWER OF CRAFTFULNESS

Not only is crafting an enjoyable, satisfying hobby – research shows that, when done regularly, craft activities can improve mental health as well as increase relaxation. And that's because loosing yourself in the detail of crafting is a natural form of mindfulness. Craftfulness, as it's popularly called, helps you achieve what Hungarian psychologist Mihaly Csikszentmihalyi called 'flow' where you're totally absorbed in your activity whether it's skiing or mending a shirt. To achieve flow, the psychologist believed there needed to be several factors in place – having a goal and set of rules; concentrating on the task at hand; merging awareness with your action; and choosing a project that requires skill and gives you feedback. As you can see, crafting fits the bill perfectly.

Getting lost in the beauty of a landscape you're painting or feeling the sensation of clay against your hands as you sculpt, keeps you fully absorbed in the moment and everyday worries melt away. If you struggle to clear your mind, crafting is an easy short cut to a mediation.

MAKE AND MEND

Crafting can bring a wealth of health benefits. Using your hands and brain together has been shown to encourage neural connections in the brain that can help combat depression. It gives you a sense of achievement as well as boosting memory and focus. It also helps you get in touch with who you really are. 'Creativity is an intrinsic part of our human-ness,' say Rosemary Davidson and Arzu Tahsin authors of the book *Craftfulness* (Quercus, £12.99). And, they add, beginning a new crafting project or learning a new skill where you need to make creative decisions can help your growth in everyday life.

BE CREATIVE

+ Swap watching TV for an adult colouring book.
+ Take a mindful walk, snapping photos of your observations.
+ Build a lego creation or complete a jigsaw puzzle.
+ Make a scrapbook or photo album.
+ If you can knit or sew, try following a pattern.
+ Teach yourself a new creative skill such as calligraphy.

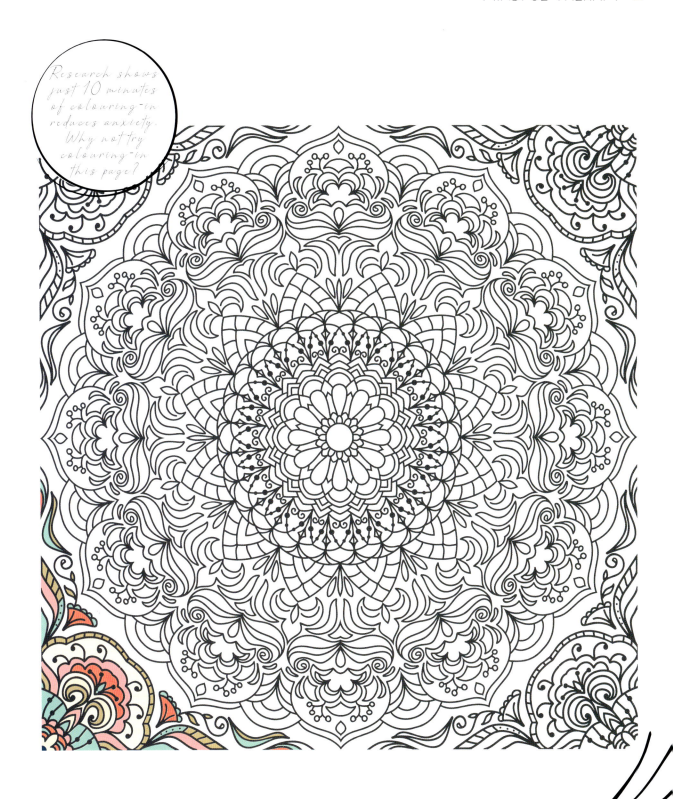

Research shows just 10 minutes of colouring-in reduces anxiety. Why not try colouring-in this page?

CREATE A VISION BOARD

Make your dreams reality with a mindfulness mood board

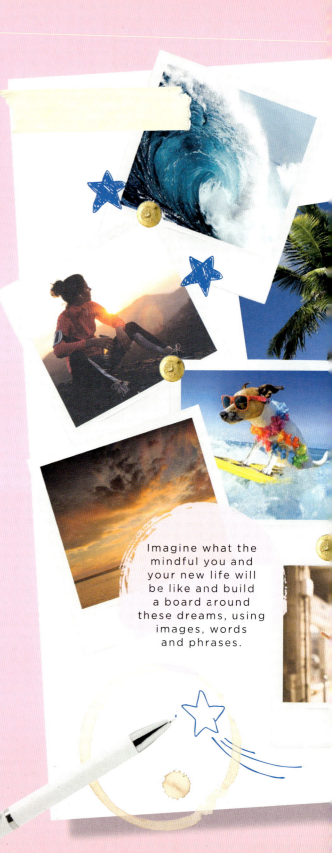

Not a natural artist? Being creative is not just about being able to draw or paint. What makes something creative is its expression of you. And the most important creation is, of course, your life. When you use nature and spirit to fuel this creation, you have powerful tools at tip of your fingers.

TRY THIS

To discover what will make your heart and soul sing, sometimes you have to bypass your conscious mind. Images often speak directly to your subconscious, so make a vision board by collecting inspiring images, and place them somewhere you'll see them every day. To help bypass your logical left brain, skip Google and lay out a selection of old magazines and other images in front of you, relax and choose any pictures you feel drawn too.

Imagine what the mindful you and your new life will be like and build a board around these dreams, using images, words and phrases.

WHAT YOU NEED

Poster board, glue stick, old magazines, photos and scissors.

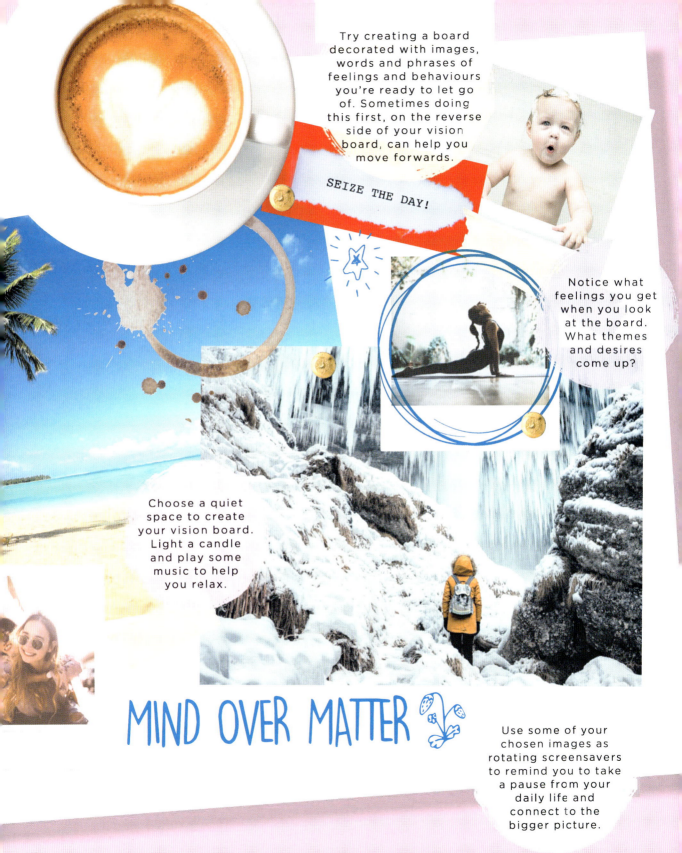

Try creating a board decorated with images, words and phrases of feelings and behaviours you're ready to let go of. Sometimes doing this first, on the reverse side of your vision board, can help you move forwards.

SEIZE THE DAY!

Notice what feelings you get when you look at the board. What themes and desires come up?

Choose a quiet space to create your vision board. Light a candle and play some music to help you relax.

MIND OVER MATTER

Use some of your chosen images as rotating screensavers to remind you to take a pause from your daily life and connect to the bigger picture.

BE GRATEFUL

Want to boost your happiness?
It's time to thank your blessings

Gratitude is a hot topic these days. We're told to make gratitude lists and feel thankful. But does practising gratitude really work? The short answer is yes. First, it can improve physical health. A University of Connecticut study of people who had suffered a heart attack found that those who saw benefits in their experience – such as being more grateful for, and appreciative of, life – had a lower risk of having another heart attack. Gratitude can help mental health too. Positive psychologists have found that people who express gratitude tend to be more optimistic and healthy than those who don't. Gratitude can lower anxiety and depression, lead to more satisfying relationships and better sleep. It can also spread good karma: if we express gratitude to other people, they're more likely to behave more generously to us and others. Convinced? Try these tips for feeling more thankful.

1. Thank everyone
Make an effort to thank everyone who does something for you, no matter how small – from another driver letting you pass first, to a colleague who makes you a cup of tea.

2. Share your positive feeling

Tell someone you find difficult how much you value them, whether it's the colleague who's always talking down to you or your needy friend. Be specific: give three reasons why you appreciate them so much. Gratitude strengthens bonds, showing a person they matter more to you than they realised.

3. Go public

ANNOUNCE YOUR PLANS TO BE MORE GRATEFUL. SHARE WITH YOUR FRIENDS ON SOCIAL MEDIA THE THINGS YOU FEEL GRATEFUL FOR. IN TIME, YOU WILL NOTICE YOU HAVE A BRIGHTER OUTLOOK AND THIS MAY RUB OFF ON YOUR FRIENDS TOO.

4. Make your inner voice more grateful

We all have an inner monologue going on and we often respond to it in subtle ways. If your inner voice is downbeat and negative, your mood will be low. Give your inner voice a more appreciative tone and your mood will lift, allowing for better actions and interactions with others.

PUT A NOTE OF GRATITUDE ON YOUR MIRROR SO YOU BEGIN THE DAY WITH A GOOD ATTITUDE. OR TRY A GRATITUDE APP ON YOUR PHONE AND CREATE SLIDE SHOWS WHEN YOU NEED A REMINDER OF HOW GOOD LIFE IS.

6. Have a gratitude buddy

This can help you keep going until gratitude becomes a habit. Find someone else who wants to practise gratitude – you could make gratitude lists every week and email them to each other. Hearing another's list can help you feel more grateful too.

7. Write a letter

POSITIVE PSYCHOLOGIST MARTIN SELIGMAN SUGGESTS WRITING A 300-WORD LETTER TO SOMEONE WHO HAS MADE A DIFFERENCE TO YOUR LIFE. GO INTO DETAIL; EXPLAIN HOW MUCH THEY CHANGED YOUR LIFE AND HOW. NOW, DELIVER IT IN PERSON AND READ IT TO THEM. IT WILL GIVE YOU BOTH A BOOST.

FEED YOUR SOUL

Connecting to your spirituality is proven to be one of the most effective wellness tonics. Here's how to tap in to it

Countless studies show that spiritual beliefs can boost your health. One large US study found that people who regularly go to church have improved life expectancy while another found that praying can help people cope with chronic pain. It's also known that having a faith can potentially help mental issues, such as depression, raise self esteem and aid faster recovery from illness.

But you don't have to be religious to reap the benefits. Spiritual practices unconnected to religion, such as yoga, can also boost your wellbeing by lowering stress and anxiety, increasing a sense of personal control and giving you a greater sense of wholeness, identity and self-awareness.

WHAT IS SPIRITUALITY?

Spirituality is about believing in a power that is outside the experience of your usual senses. It connects you to a wider purpose and gives you the sense that you're part of a whole. It's about finding joy with everything around you and allowing unconditional love to exist inside of you.

You don't need to go to a place of worship to practise spirituality. It can be private and personal. Meditation, yoga, walking in the countryside and reflecting on your connection with nature can all help you tap into your spiritual side. Here are some ideas to try.

1 BREATHE
Learn to meditate (see page 52). For many people, this is the first step to tapping into their spirituality.

3 MAKE A SPECIAL PLACE
Create a spiritual environment. Try making a shrine in a quiet spot of your house, decorated with precious possessions or photographs, where you can sit and contemplate. Try burning frankincense essential oil, which is known for its spiritual properties.

5 REACH OUT
The community aspect of religion is thought to be one of its most healing benefits. Try getting involved in a local project or charity.

2 PROTECT YOUR TIME
Connect with nature. Relax and soak up the richness of nature and its ability just to be alive.

4 BE MUSICAL
Singing can cut stress and lower blood pressure. So why not join a choir for the sheer joy of hearing other people's voices? Even if you're not creating music yourself, just listening helps you feel uplifted.

6 GET MOVING
Try soulful exercise. Working out can be a spiritual experience. The best activities for this purpose are those you don't have to concentrate too much on, such as swimming, dancing and hiking.

Day 25

TRY SOME MIRROR WORK. BEFORE YOUR SHOWER OR BATH, TAKE FIVE MINUTES TO LOOK AT YOURSELF, NAKED, IN THE MIRROR. OBSERVE YOUR FACE AND BODY WITHOUT JUDGEMENT. THIS IS A TRICKY ONE AS WE'RE SO CONDITIONED INTO THINKING ABOUT DIFFERENT PARTS OF OUR BODY AS 'GOOD' OR 'BAD' — BUT THIS EXERCISE IS ABOUT MINDFUL ACCEPTANCE OF YOURSELF JUST AS YOU ARE. LOOK CAREFULLY AT EVERY INCH OF YOUR BODY, NOTICING DETAILS SUCH AS MOLES, FRECKLES AND FOLDS OF SKIN. EVERY TIME A CRITICAL THOUGHT SWIMS INTO YOUR MIND, THANK IT, AND LET IT GO.

HOW I FELT

TODAY'S MINDFUL MOMENTS

Day 26

HAVE A MINDFUL EVENING ROUTINE. RATHER THAN WATCHING TELLY, THEN FLOPPING INTO BED, SPEND HALF AN HOUR UNWINDING. HAVE A RELAXING BATH WITH SOME SOOTHING LAVENDER OIL AND TAKE YOUR TIME WASHING, NOTICING THE FEELING OF YOUR HANDS ON YOUR SKIN AND THE WARM WATER AGAINST YOUR BODY. MAKE YOURSELF A CUP OF CALMING VALERIAN TEA AND SIP IT SLOWLY WITH YOUR EYES CLOSED, SAVOURING THE FLAVOUR AND FEELING THE HEAT OF THE TEA AS IT PASSES YOUR MOUTH AND THROAT. LISTEN TO SOME CALMING CLASSICAL MUSIC IN YOUR BEDROOM AS YOU PREPARE TO FALL ASLEEP.

HOW I FELT

TODAY'S MINDFUL MOMENTS

Sea

Day 27

NOTICE TRANSITIONS. TODAY, WHENEVER YOU COME IN FROM THE COLD AND DARK OUTSIDE, BE MINDFUL OF THE CHANGE WHEN YOU MOVE INDOORS. NOTICE THE WARMTH, THE LIGHT, AND THE WAY YOUR BODY FEELS AS YOU GO INSIDE. CONVERSELY, WHEN YOU GO OUT, BE FULLY AWARE OF THE BRIGHTNESS, COLDER TEMPERATURES AND DIFFERENT SOUNDS AS YOU MOVE FROM THE INSIDE TO THE OUTSIDE. NOTICE THE THOUGHTS THAT COME AND GO AS YOU MOVE INTO DIFFERENT ENVIRONMENTS, AND ALL THE CHANGES IN YOUR BODY'S REACTIONS. KEEP DOING THIS AND YOU'LL GAIN A NEW APPRECIATION OF CHANGE.

HOW I FELT

TODAY'S MINDFUL MOMENTS

Day 28

INCREASE YOUR MEDITATION TIME. NOW YOU'VE BEEN MEDITATING FOR FIVE MINUTES A DAY, TRY RAISING IT TO 10 MINUTES. THIS WILL GIVE YOU A MORE IN-DEPTH EXPERIENCE OF MINDFULNESS MEDITATION AND YOU SHOULD QUICKLY NOTICE THE DIFFERENCE IT MAKES TO YOUR DAY AND YOUR STRESS LEVELS. FOLLOW EXACTLY THE SAME PRINCIPLES — SIMPLY FOCUS ON YOUR BREATHING AND CONTINUE TO BRING YOUR MIND BACK TO THE MOMENT BUT KEEP GOING FOR 10 MINUTES — AND CONTINUE TO BUILD UP THE MINUTES.

HOW I FELT

TODAY'S MINDFUL MOMENTS

DIRECTORY

EQUIPMENT

Gaiam
Gaiam.com

Ty Burhoe & Tala Records
tyburhoe.com

Yoga Matters
yogamatters.com

INSTRUCTION

Be Mindful
bemindful.co.uk

EkhartYoga
ekhartyoga.com

Harley Therapy
harleytherapy.co.uk

Jack Kornfield
jackkornfield.com

London Meditation Centre
londonmeditationcentre.com

Tara Brach
tarabrach.com

Sharon Salzberg
sharonsalzberg.com

Uz Afzal
beherebreathe.co.uk

Will Williams
willwilliamsmeditation.co.uk

BOOKS

The Miracle of Mindfulness,
Thich Nhat Hanh
(Rider, £8.99)

*Where You Go, There
You Are*, Jon Kabat-Zinn
(Piatkus, £13.99)

*Bringing Home the Dharma:
Awakening Right Where
You Are*, Jack Kornfield
(Shambhala Publications
Inc, £13.99)

*Real Happiness: The
Power of Meditation*,
Sharon Salzburg
(Workman Publishing, £11.55)

*100 Mindfulness Meditations:
The Ultimate Collection of
Inspiring Daily Practices*,
Neil Seligman
(Conscious House, £12.99)

*Mindfulness for
Children*, Uz Afzal
(Kyle Books, £14.99)

*Run For Your Life – Mindful
Running for a Happy Life*,
William Pullen
(Penguin Life, £9.99)

Mindfulness @ Work,
Anna Black
(Cico Books, £12.99)

APPS

Aura
aurahealth.io

Calm
Calm.com

Headspace
Headspace.com

Insight Timer
insighttimer.com

Silatha
silatha.com

THE EXPERTS

With thanks to the experts who have contributed to this book

NEIL SELIGMAN

(*Prepare to practise*, p50; *Musical healing*, p64)

Neil Seligman is a leading mindfulness expert, author and speaker with CEOs, global firms and celebrities among his clients. He is author of the book *100 Mindfulness Meditations: The Ultimate Collection of Inspiring Daily Practices* (Conscious House, £12.99). It was meeting a reiki master while working at a children's summer camp as a student, that set Neil on a journey to discover the world of inner consciousness. After completing a master's in reiki, Neil left behind his career as star barrister to follow a more spiritual path and founded The Conscious Professional, a corporate consultancy through which Neil shares his wisdom on mindfulness and transformation around the world. Visit neilseligman.com

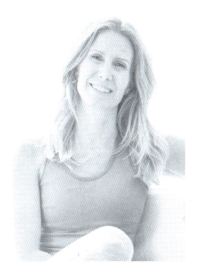

ESTHER EKHART & EKHARTYOGA

(*Stretch & Soothe*, p98)

Esther Ekhart has taught yoga internationally for over 20 years. EkhartYoga was born from Esther's dream to share the love of yoga, and today thousands of students worldwide practise online yoga and meditation through the channel. With more than 3,000 classes in different styles guided by over 40 world-class teachers, it's Europe's biggest online studio. Esther has thousands of students following her online classes, where she teaches stronger yoga styles including Vinyasa Flow and Hatha as well as slower practices including Yin yoga, meditation and restorative yoga, which allow you to 'drop in' and get to know yourself better. Creating positive transformation through yoga remains at the heart of everything EkhartYoga does. Join at ekhartyoga.com; FB: @EstherEkhart; IG: @estherekhart.yoga

WILLIAM PULLEN

(*On the run*, p94)

William Pullen is a psychotherapist registered with the British Association for Counselling and Psychotherapy. He practices Integrative therapy and specialises in the treatment of depression, anxiety and self esteem problems. He developed Dynamic Running Therapy, which combines movement with traditional talk therapy and the outdoor environment. He is author of *Run for Your Life - Mindful Running for a Happy Life* (Penguin Life, £9.99). Visit dynamicrunningtherapy.co.uk

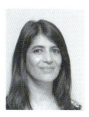

UZ AFZAL

(*Mindfulness for kids*, p80)

Uz Afzal has worked in education for 20 years. She is a Mindfulness Based Stress Reduction teacher, is trained in Paws B and Dot B Mindfulness in Schools Programme and in teaching The Mindful Schools Curriculum. Uz was selected to become a consultant for Goldie Hawn's MindUP Programme. She is author of *Mindfulness for Children* (Kyle Books, £14.99). Visit beherebreathe.co.uk

VERONIEK VERMEULEN

(*The power of journaling*, p32)

Founder of Silatha, Veroniek Vermeulen discovered the power of mindfulness while at a meditation retreat in Nepal during a career break. After continuing her mindfulness training, Veroniek left behind the corporate world and set up Silatha which creates handcrafted jewellery based around the dorje (an ancient meditation symbol) made with gemstones that align with an inner quality to be nutured. Each piece of jewellery comes with the Silatha Meditation Course App which offers a series of guided meditations over 21 days. Visit silatha.com

Photograph of William Pullen: Angelo Valentino

ENJOY THE JOURNEY

We hope you've enjoyed your journey into mindfulness. Hopefully by now, you've already had a taste of the incredible calm and ease it can bring you. You now have all the knowledge and skills you need to bring mindfulness practice into your life and reap its transformative powers. And the more you use the practices in this book, the more benefits you'll enjoy.

Use *The Mindfulness Workbook* and 28-day Journal as a reminder and guide as you continue your mindfulness journey. Perhaps you feel inspired to do some further study, sign up for a meditation class or try some mindful exercise? Whatever else is happening in your life, giving yourself a moment to connect to your breath and return to your inner truth is all you need to live a happier, richer life.

Remember, this is just the beginning...

'Every morning we are born again. What we do today is what matters most'

BUDDHA

THE
MINDFULNESS
WORKBOOK

Editor Mary Comber
Art Director Lucy Pinto
Chief Sub-editor Sheila Reid
Writers Mary Comber, Charlotte Haigh, Eve Boggenpoel

With thanks to: Uz Afzal, Esther Ekhart, William Pullen,
Neil Seligman, Veroniek Vermeulen

Publisher Steven O'Hara
Publishing Director Dan Savage
Marketing Manager Charlotte Park
Commercial Director Nigel Hole

Printed by William Gibbons & Sons, Wolverhampton

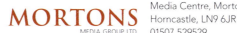

Published by Mortons Media Group Ltd,
Media Centre, Morton Way,
Horncastle, LN9 6JR
01507 529529

The Mindfulness Workbook ISBN 9781911639145

While every care was taken during the production of this Bookazine, the publishers cannot be held responsible for the accuracy of the information or any consequence arising from it. Mortons Media Group takes on responsibility for the companies advertising in this Bookazine. The paper used within this Bookazine is produced from sustainable fibre, manufactured by mills with a valid chain of custody.

The health and fitness information presented in this book is an educational resource and is not intended as a substitute for medical advice. Consult your doctor or healthcare professional before performing any of the exercises described in this book or any other exercise programme, particularly if you are pregnant, or if you are elderly or have chronic or recurring medical conditions. Do not attempt any of the exercises while under the influence of alcohol or drugs.

Discontinue any exercise that causes you pain or severe discomfort and consult a medical expert.
Neither the author of the information nor the producer nor distributors of such information make
any warranty of any kind in regard to the content of the information presented in this book.

This magazine is published under license from and with the permission of Dennis Publishing Limited. All rights in the material and the title and trademark of this magazine belong to Dennis Publishing Limited absolutely and may not be reproduced, whether in whole or in part, without its prior consent.

'Live the actual moment.
Only this moment
is life'

THICH NHAT HANH